PENGUIN BOOKS

COVID-19: A BLACK COMEDY OF EMOTIONAL INTELLIGENCE

Born in 1976, Natasha is a creative communications specialist with 19 years in education, creative arts and the media industry. Her work was instrumental in creating the communicative arts curriculum design for Taylors' Design School under the School of Architecture, Building and Design at Taylor's University from 2004-2010. She also designed and taught the Performing Arts module at Taylor's School of Communication for over 6 years that paved the way for its first Performing Arts Conservatory launched in 2019. A signature of her work fuses performative, visual and fine arts with strong advocacy on cultural preservation and cross-culture literacy, as powerful expressive and therapeutic tools having collaborated with Kakiseni, the Malaysian Invention & Design Society and UNESCO under the Venezuelan embassy.

Her work under the BAC Education Group from 2014-2019 includes spearheading IACT College with a series of high-impact industry projects centred on social development targeting marginalized communities and controversial issues such as LGBT, rare diseases and Humanitarian work creating a strong alliance with the Make It Right Movement (MIRM), Mercy Malaysia and SEED Foundation. Her role includes redesigning the entity's communication curriculum programmes to facilitate increased youth employability and to promote innovative teaching and learning.

Natasha was part of the UNICEF team with HELP University in 2006 to conduct two meaningful research projects: the traumatic effects of the 2004 Aceh tsunami on children and a nationwide research on bullying across Malaysian schools. Her exposure in these areas intensified her passion to travel across the country to create, provide and promote workshops on creative pedagogy based on trauma, emotional constructs and performative design.

In 2019 Natasha served as COO at Tandemic, a regional innovation firm specialising in Design Thinking (DT) training and Agile management, consultancy on innovation lab work, and social research. Her portfolio covered business development and strategy, and as a DT trainer with clients such as MyXpats, CIMB, UOB FinLab, Coca-Cola, TalentCorp, Penang Council, and Novo Nordisk.

Natasha was formerly the CEO of a social impact batik company that produces batik textile Gahara focusing on its domestic and international corporate strategy; Executive Committee member of the Malaysia Craft Council in pushing for education on and advocacy in artisanal representation for local arts and crafts; Industry Advisor for the Malaysian Institute of Architects (PAM). Natasha is currently pursuing her doctorate in Business Administration specializing in the areas of organizational behaviour, design and transformational leadership. Natasha's current work is in the European Union delving into green technology to address circular fashion and improve textile processing.

COVID-19: A Black Comedy of Emotional Intelligence

A Book Written During

Quarantine

by

Natasha MH

PENGUIN BOOKS

An imprint of Penguin Random House

PENGUIN BOOKS

USA | Canada | UK | Ireland | Australia
New Zealand | India | South Africa | China | Southeast Asia

Penguin Books is part of the Penguin Random House group of companies
whose addresses can be found at global.penguinrandomhouse.com

Published by Penguin Random House SEA Pte Ltd
9, Changi South Street 3, Level 08-01,
Singapore 486361

Penguin
Random House
SEA

First published in Penguin Books by Penguin Random House SEA 2021
Copyright © Natasha MH 2021

ISBN 9789814954419

Typeset in Adobe Garamond Pro by MAP Systems, Bangalore, India

www.penguin.sg

Pandora's Box has been opened

The pandemic crisis of 2020 is not showing us that our lives are irrevocably damaged. On the contrary, it reminds us of our role towards humanity, that some areas may have been neglected and systems need to be upgraded.

From weak healthcare systems, poor leadership, to the frailty of human communication, *COVID-19: A Black Comedy of Emotional Intelligence* is both a social satire and a reflection exercise towards becoming a more engaged citizen of the world after the virus turned the world upside down. So much was conveyed from mainstream media, social media, skeptics and conspiracy theorists alike which rose to the surface like crema, an interesting tapestry of reexamining life as how we know it. A pandemic united the world, many agreed to disagree on how the future of the planet ought to be handled. Halting capitalism cleaned oceans and cleared the atmosphere, people saw ugly truths of their governments with their backhanded policies. But will life ever be the same again? It isn't just a story about the world in action but also about countries and their *inaction*. And where do we go from here?

A book written during quarantine, a lot of the insights are inspired by writings on Heart Intelligence (HQ) designed to guide the reader towards Alvin Toffler's dictum of 'Learning, Unlearning and Relearning'. Readers can benefit from the compilation of facts and sardonic approach. Each chapter ends with insights and suggestions for personal reflection.

Written from March 2020 to June 2021

What is this book about? My friend asked.

Good question. I ask this myself every morning when I wake up.

Some days the words come easy, with clarity. Some days it gets fuzzy. Some days I question all that I've considered.

And that was how it felt during the COVID-19 lockdown.

Some days you were up. Some days down. Some days with joy, some days with doubts. Many days with anxiety coalesced by an ongoing stream of frustration.

This book is about surviving as it is about being.

It's also about democracy. About democracy of self, sanity and state.

Most important of all, it's about learning. Quarantine gave us (plenty) time to reflect.

I turned forty-four when COVID-19 started. A week after my birthday, we went into lockdown (Movement Control Order known as MCO).

I turned forty-five and was in another lockdown (MCO 2.0).

In May 2021 we entered MCO 3.0.

In between the months, seasons passed, the economy crashed like another Great Depression, jobs created in the past seventy years were lost, and many of my childhood celebrities died.

Even a year on, experts worldwide are still stymied by the virus asking, what, and how?

It seems ironic, that in movies, humans always seemed to be brilliant in saving the planet from natural disasters. We'd come up with all sorts of weapons, expertise and life-saving mechanisms and superheroes. We have tiers of intelligences from military to artificial, yet when the real world came into crisis by an unseen assailant brought upon by biology, not aliens from outer space, the world's best and brightest struggled to connect the dots.

To the best of my ability during distressing times, this book is about making sense of a world that no longer makes any sense, yet I am determined to survive it.

Franz Werfel wrote: '*Thirst is the surest proof for the existence of water.*' I am determined to see my favourite ocean, the Mediterranean, once more when the borders reopen. With the people that I love. It's not about when, it's the fact that I will.

And right now, the only weapon I've got to arm myself with, is my emotional intelligence.

Not just mine, but all of ours.

Table of Contents

Prologue

The writing of this book owes gratitude to Michelle Obama and Anne Frank. They sowed the seeds of thought which led to a string of chapters.

It was March and the first lockdown was issued. The year is 2020. It sounds like an opening from an Aldous Huxley novel. Ironic. Identical keywords and concepts. Totalitarianism. New World Order. Power and control. Much has yet to come.

A 2019 coronavirus disease (shortened to COVID-19) has spiralled out of control from a sprawling city named Wuhan in China, and has done the unthinkable: crossed international borders.

Defined as an illness caused by a novel coronavirus called severe acute respiratory syndrome coronavirus 2 (SARS-CoV-2; formerly called 2019-nCoV), which was first identified amid an outbreak of respiratory disease, its genesis remains a mystery more than a year later.

Initially accused of being transmitted from bats to humans, there are rising suspicions that it's a manmade biological hazard that leaked out of a lab.

According to reports such as Medscape, presentations of COVID-19 range from 'asymptomatic/mild symptoms to severe illness and mortality. Symptoms may develop two days to two weeks after exposure to the virus. A pooled analysis of 181 confirmed cases of COVID-19 outside Wuhan, China, found the mean incubation period to be 5.1 days and that 97.5 per cent of individuals who developed symptoms did so within 11.5 days of infection.'

The Chinese Centre for Disease Control and Prevention (CDC) issued a recommendation that the general public, even those without symptoms, should begin wearing face coverings in public settings where social distancing measures are difficult to maintain to abate the spread of COVID-19. The CDC had postulated that this situation could result in large numbers of patients requiring medical care concurrently, resulting in overloaded public health and healthcare systems and, potentially, elevated rates of hospitalization and deaths. The CDC advised that nonpharmaceutical interventions (NPIs) are the most important response strategies for delaying viral spread and reducing disease impact. Unfortunately, these concerns have been proven accurate.

> The feasibility and implications suppression and mitigation strategies have been rigorously analysed and are being encouraged or enforced by many governments to slow or halt viral transmission. Population-wide social distancing plus other interventions (eg, home self-isolation, school and business closures) are strongly advised. These policies may be required for long periods to avoid rebound viral transmission.

On March 11, the World Health Organization (WHO) declared COVID-19 a pandemic. There were talks of a zombie apocalypse.

My birthday had passed four days earlier. After watching the Malaysian Prime Minister Muhyiddin Yassin's broadcast on television regarding the Movement Control Order (MCO) I asked myself what's next? What's next for lunch, what's next for work, what's next for life?

Like many others around the world in a time of crisis and confusion, restricted to our homes, I resorted to Youtube to kill time. Time is going to be plenty in our hands from now on. Earlier en route to my room I had passed my father's bookshelf and saw Michelle Obama's book *Becoming* which my mother received as a gift earlier in November 2019. In an attempt to skip reading the book, on a whim I typed 'Michelle Obama' on my laptop in the search box and watched the first few links that appeared. To amuse myself, I thought, 'Whatever these videos reveal, it will be a guide.' Follow the esoteric compass.

I clicked on a random link. In an interview with Jimmy Kimmel, Michelle was asked about her early days as FLOTUS (First Lady of the United States). What were your days like? Kimmel asked. Mrs Obama replied, 'I was given a to-do list.

'The President's wife is given a list on what she needs to accomplish tailored for the First Lady,' she recalled. 'The list included writing a book.'

The Magician tarot card flashed in my mind. *Crash boom bang*

Michelle Obama continued, 'Honestly, I struggled on what to write. In the end I decided to write about the things I'm often asked, to go deeper into the experiences that shaped me towards being FLOTUS.'

As a form of practice, there were transcripts of what the First Lady had done (and must be recorded) at the White House. 'Weeks and events go by so fast it helped to document what had happened,' the FLOTUS explained. 'And there were those popular curious topics like living in the White House, raising a family under constant watch, and being married to one of the world's most charismatic leaders. The fact that they were frequently asked meant it was significant to people.'

Michelle Obama didn't expect the book to take off the way it did. It became the bestselling book of 2018. 'To write a book was an expectation for me as the wife of the President. It was on the list and so I did it.'

And that was my epiphany. The fact FLOTUS just did it, like an obedient student completing an assignment sans any complaints. My admiration for her increased threefold almost immediately. I scribbled a '*How to Survive COVID*' list. *Item #1: Be like Michelle Obama and write a book*. Taking a cue from Michelle, I thought of the significance of the day. There was COVID-19, a novel virus, and there was us, the populace, confined to our homes, unsure of the future. The fate of our lives were placed in the hands of elected global leaders, medical and health experts while everything else from businesses, shopping centres to learning institutions had been suspended.

Despite the virus being unlettered to us, toilet rolls were flying off supermarket shelves. It made repeated headlines. *So why do people panic buy toilet rolls in times of crisis?* It made no sense.

As the days unfolded it was not just the toilet rolls.

In Malaysia, where I live, bread was flying off shelves. Since time immemorial in the Southeast Asian basin, our staple food has been rice. While, oddly, rice was in steady supply, the pandemic had turned the locals French towards pastries. One household brand Gardenia was pressured to produce more bread since they rolled their first loaf in 1986. It became a joke that rational everyday folks were chasing

Gardenia bread trucks. Breadmakers became popular on Shopee and suddenly even my sisters-in-law were making focaccia, and my friends sourdough buns. There was an influx of bake posts on social media like the new porn.

> At first I was consumed by a conspiracy theory of my own. Without triggering users' awareness, the COVID-19 construction was a global-scale exercise on prediction analysis, seeing government's actions and inactions. It was an opportunity to observe how nations conducted respective grid searches on themselves to process and survive the pandemic, and which ones possessed the most crippled defence systems. On a larger perspective, it wasn't about the fragility of our immune or healthcare systems, but of countries, ruling governments and ALL their systems. COVID-19 is a beta testing programme in the midst of iterations, awaiting an alpha release.

Over the months that followed, from headlines to headlines I came to see the world in a very different way. Indeed the world was far from perfect. Systemically broken, corrupted and abused. But I also saw new light in the human spirit. Our fight for survival in captivity, armed with only words exchanged on screens, faces hidden behind masks on the streets. There were moments, incidents and breaking news that had to be written about. Some were domestic, others abroad. Yet, all had a connective tissue. There are stories of leadership, stories for mental dexterity, and reflections on case studies that contemplate the problems and dilemmas that we are facing.

Germaine Greer, an Australian writer and public intellectual regarded as one of the major voices of the radical feminist movement in the later half of the twentieth century writes, 'Perhaps catastrophe is the natural human environment, and even though we spend a good deal of energy trying to get away from it, we are programmed for survival amid catastrophe.'

I saw the relevance of writing this book as a way to grasp my own sanity and to create equilibrium at a unique time where the world was losing its balance. Little did I know I was going to lose mine on several occasions. In his book *Social Intelligence: The New Science of Human Relationships* author and science journalist Daniel Goleman writes:

> Self-absorption in all its forms kills empathy, let alone compassion. When we focus on ourselves, our world contracts as our problems and preoccupations loom large. But when we focus on others, our world expands. Our own problems drift to the periphery of the mind and so seem smaller, and we increase our capacity for connection - or compassionate action.

I thought perhaps a healthy outlet was to journal what was happening in and around the world rather than to dwell on my own misery while licking self-pity. As Aristotle wrote in *The Nicomachean Ethics*: 'Anyone can become angry—that is easy. But to be angry with the right person, to the right degree, at the right time, for the right purpose, and in the right way—this is not easy.'

Indeed, who am I to be angry for the pain of being locked up for my own good?

Marcus Aurelius had this to say millennia ago about pain: 'Pain is not due to the thing itself, but to your estimate of it, and that you have the power to revoke at any moment.' Emotional intelligence is what will save us all from this wretched existence of a pandemic.

Perhaps this can be an adventure

In times of adversity, people often reveal their fears, hopes, strengths and frailties. But I didn't want to be swept away by the norm. I wasn't making bread, craving bread or chasing bread trucks. I also didn't buy a Thermomix, had no intention of becoming an overnight indoor gardener, and binge on online shopping.

Enduring COVID-19 like everyone else, I had my own significant experiences. Like the practice at the White House, I decided that what I observed, I will document. Assuming we keep this book in a time capsule in the event another global outbreak occurs, perhaps a bigger catastrophe, this book can offer relief. As Anne Frank wrote in the secret annex her father built for protection where she was confined for two years during the Nazi invasion, 'I keep my ideals, because in spite of everything I still believe that people are really good at heart. How wonderful it is that nobody needs to wait a single moment before starting to improve the world. Think of all the beauty still left around you and be happy.'

Frank was not the only one who survived confinement through writing. Turns out many did. The Minister of Education of the Dutch government, after fleeing to England, made an appeal on Radio Orange to hold on to war diaries and documents so that it would be clear after the war what they all had experienced during the German occupation.

It was upon hearing this announcement that Anne was inspired to publish a book after the war about her time in hiding. She also came up with a title: *Het Achterhuis*, or The Secret Annex. She started working on this project on 20 May 1944. She describes the period from 12 June 1942 to 29 March 1944. In those months Anne wrote around 50,000 words, filling more than 215 sheets of paper. Though sadly Anne was captured and died in the Bergen-Belsen concentration camp, it is her writing that motivates us to survive hard times. Writing was Anne's own way to escape, to reflect and to hold on. She describes, writing in her diary, 'The nicest part is being able to write down all my thoughts and feelings; otherwise, I'd absolutely suffocate.'

Stories of confinement, like chronicles of war, are critical to the growth of human survival. When Sigmund Freud wrote the *Interpretations of Dreams* in 1899 to suggest forms of subliminal leakages that influence our awakened behaviour, people scoffed at its lack of scientific basis. How can we understand what cannot be measured? Significance of dreams? Today, Freud's psychology is at the heart of all disciplines, from quantum physics, healthcare, architecture, through to hostage crisis negotiation and criminal profiling. Frank's diary gave us perspective on human survival from a young girl who matured and blossomed on faith, hope and optimism at a time when someone her age today may take her own life soaked in medication, alcohol and depression. The common thread is social psychology. Just like how Freud's work becomes a crucial underpinning to how we understand modern life, stories of struggles written during times of crises help navigate us for survival.

We may not be at war but our emotional intelligence is at battle due to today's social complexities. COVID-19 upends it all and puts us on a tailspin.

On day 761 in hiding, Anne wrote her last entry. Describing herself as 'a bundle of contradictions,' she wrote: 'As I've told you many times, I'm split in two. One side contains my exuberant cheerfulness, my flippancy, my joy in life and, above all, my ability to appreciate the lighter side of things.'

When asked, what would she tell her pre-White House self in a *Good Morning America* segment, Michelle Obama describes, 'It is going to be hard, I realized I would have to earn my grace. And with all the comments and criticism I received, most bitter is the experience of people taking over my voice. I needed to own that. Own my own voice.'

And so I decided, this book is a voice—my voice, curiosity, warts and all—among many in the days of corona.

The pandemic woke me up from a reverie and into a new reality, and rightfully so. The following chapters are stories written during the three lockdowns issued by the government of Malaysia from March 2020 to June 2021. Preferring to call them reflections and thought pieces with no intention to preach, they became a smorgasbord of eclectic discourse connected to philosophy, psychology, business, leadership and a gamut of ideology that underpins our thoughts and social experiences. From Freud, Goleman, Kissinger, the US presidential election, Malaysian politics, freedom of speech, history, racism, to growth mindset, COVID-19 was no longer about a medical emergency. Each chapter narrates a significant human event, be it bleak or bright, that connects us to one another despite circumstances that may seem otherwise. In the final analysis, I realized I had written a book for the future generation. I hope the message within would inspire a call to action so tomorrow will be better than today.

H.G. Wells would have gone 'I told you so'

Statistics define disaster
We panic at the thought of impact
Meteorologists say it's not a big deal
If a tree falls in the forest and no one hears, does it count?

These were the thoughts of confusion as a pandemic outbreak was declared worldwide.

All that keeps racing through my mind in the early days of 2020 leading into March are the four statements, when headlines were colliding with the staggering infection rates against an unknown assailant. It felt like being in an echo chamber as news after news kept mentioning a world going into strict and extended lockdowns. *Against a flu? How bad is this thing? And the entire world?*

Not since 11 September 2001 did the world stand fastened to their news portals as American Airlines Flight 11 and United Airlines Flight 175, crashed into the North and South Towers, respectively, of the World Trade Center complex in Lower Manhattan. Within an hour and forty-two minutes, both of the 110-storey towers collapsed. Debris and the resulting fires caused a partial or complete collapse of all other buildings in the World Trade Center complex, including the forty-seven storey 7 World Trade Center tower, as well as significant damage to ten other large surrounding structures. A third plane crashed into the Pentagon, and a fourth towards Washington D.C. but crashed in a township in Pennsylvania. The attacks resulted in 2,977 fatalities, over 25,000 injuries, and substantial long-term health consequences, in addition to at least $10 billion in infrastructure and property damage. It is the deadliest terrorist attack in human history.

'But that's America's problem,' the rest of the world said. Once the shock had dissipated, we were able to remove ourselves from the story and head back to our normal lives.

Although the statistics for the 9/11 attack remain dubious up till today, the fact remains that the rest of the world wished the people of the United States their condolences and was unaffected by its aftermath. Eventually, all airport security loosened their grip and flying felt safe again.

Today, this is different.

This is like *The War of the Worlds*. Indeed, we have been invaded by aliens.

We can't see our attackers. This coronavirus is out for everyone including those who had hijacked the planes of 9/11, the Wahhabi terrorist group Al-Qaeda. The world is at the mercy of a possible biological warfare. Who is behind it? Why are searches on people like Bill Gates popular all of a sudden? Agenda 21? A depopulation conspiracy?

Hang on a minute, Bill Gates? Isn't he a tech geek? Are we looking at this correctly?

Something is rotten in the state of Denmark.

It started out like any other year

If there is one certainty, we are not walking out of this Corona episode the same people we walked in. And that is perhaps the beauty of it. Reporting from Malaysia under a Movement Controlled Order issued from 18 March to 14 April. First journal entry:

On 31 December 2019 in Wuhan, China, cases of pneumonia with unknown aetiology were reported to the WHO China country office. While the rest of the world toasted to the new year, by 3 January 2020 cases grew to forty-four case-patients raising more questions and barely any answers. Skip forward to WHO situation report sixty-two; on 21 March 2020 the virus was detected as a novel coronavirus (later termed as COVID-19) and had infected 292,142 people with 12,784 deaths. China issued a total lockdown, South Korea monitored its citizens via mobile apps, Italy collapsed, and the United States were second to Italy with the highest number of infected cases per day, pitted against an inadequate healthcare system that they themselves did not realize was so crippled. Across the globe, a restricted movement order was issued by respective governments and people were not taking it too well. Panic shopping ensured, optimism bias grew strong and more people were still sneaking to the outdoors than staying in when authorities weren't looking. For lack of a better word, people were going apeshit. COVID-19 had raised an ugly truth: people were as resistant to being held in captivity as was the contagion relentlessly attacking people of all ages.

But I am not an epidemiologist. I am a relational systems reader, someone who studies relationships and the creative communication aspects of human connection. I probe into the areas of creativity, motivation and imagination and see how they affect human behaviour in unique situations. And here's how I process: when the movement control order (MCO) was announced here in my native country of Malaysia, my immediate response was almost like an oracle, that there will be a spike in divorce because mental health conditions such as anxiety will hit the roof, and many people will realize they don't like themselves and the people around them as much as they thought. A lockdown or quarantine will push people into corners of themselves they have been avoiding. Fourteen days are sufficient to trigger underlying conflicts even over house chores and bring out the best and the worst of ourselves. And with our shadow self comes the silver lining. People will rediscover new interests, hobbies, skills and even love. However, as a result, people will want to redesign their lives and this includes making drastic changes and leaving people, family members included, behind. Question is: are we ready for this?

We are smart but are we intelligent? As China begins to recover, numerous reports show a sharp spike in divorce applications post-coronavirus quarantine, a result of 'spending too much time together'. It sounds like a giggle but the truth cuts deeper into the iceberg of the human psyche as we begin to uncover how social distancing and quarantine makes a killer social drink, quite literally.

So what is happening, and what has this to do with design and creativity? Emotional intelligence, the root that makes us effective humans. The fact that we have emotional intelligence is critical yet we are so poor at facilitating it, especially in times of crisis.

Ironically, it is adversity that reveals our actual strength (or lack of) in being decent, being rational, being fair, being loving and being creative. It is almost like the game you play at leadership boot camps where you need to decide who gets to live and who gets to perish on an extinct planet. And right now, the skeleton key to surviving the restricted movement order, more so a lockdown, is our creative imagination. Not science, not mathematics.

In his 1995 book, *Emotional Intelligence, Why It Can Matter More Than IQ,* Daniel Goleman describes five critical units that shape our emotional intelligence (EI): self-awareness, self-regulation, motivation, empathy and social skills. And no simulation can outdo what COVID-19 has presented to us, to stay indoors and to stay put. Period. Has it been easy? Hardly.

Social media has been marvellous in providing so much data on the content being shared across the globe, proving all five units of our EI are being brutally knocked about in our cognitive hemispheres. Rants on missing out, longing for friends, anxiety caused by confined spaces, isolation surfacing feelings of abandonment, frustration in dealing with family members without adequate room for 'personal space'. Those with school-going children share tales of disappointment within themselves for not being able to play the role of teacher, coach, facilitator, nanny and parent for days on end. Parents with young children, namely toddlers, feel the strain of their parenting skills. Those who are single feel inadequate. Then there are those feeling helpless for not being able to do more to help 'those in need'. And there are those who simply cannot sit still to save their own lives which is the principal reason why the contagion has exponentially spread across towns, cities, and borders beyond control. It isn't a mere cough that spreads to others, it is that one moment of weakness when we decided to gather among friends, to run that marathon, go to that Spring Break party, to chill.

Why are we *exactly* freaking out? While the media is showing the science of the virus, social media is showing us the psychological ramification of the outbreak. While science can study the genetic sequence of the novel virus to assist pharmaceutical companies to create vaccines and to produce the reagent and equipment needed for testing, human behaviour has been a lot harder to contain and mitigate to the extent the government is threatening to use military force because we are, basically, stubborn as hell.

But there are external factors causing this emotional and behavioural fraction. Inducing this Herculean level of resistance is poor leadership. Sorely lacking is a systems leadership approach that requires empathy, social skills and maturity. In Malaysia we had a few case studies to reflect a gap in this tripartite model: when the ministry of education disallowed online learning without plausible reason and ordered students to return to their hometown as soon as the Prime Minister's office instructed citizens 'to not travel'. And while our Minister of Health was demonstrating how drinking warm water would kill the virus from the acid in our stomach, South Korea's Foreign Minister was sharing the effectiveness of their country's strategic planning using the same technology we have. And then there was the Prime Minister talking down on the citizens like a fed-up headmaster. The struggle is real, every restless Malaysian household was an echo of a restless country led by leaders who could not communicate effectively information that was meant to save lives and the confusion was disenfranchising people of transparency leading to fatalities.

And then there is the gap of information.

With the internet making people professors of opinions, the wealth of open sources create more myopic people (more specifically Whatsapp group chats) ignorant of the basics; there is no such thing as *halal* sanitizers, hoarding food exacerbates the current situation, staying in *really* save lives for as long as it requires us to be indoors, and mass congregations for prayers will not influence God's leniency on hygiene. And this gap will push the economy further to the brink of irreparable despair. From conspiracy theories to home remedies and garlic recipes to prevent infection, Facebook, Google and Twitter are wrestling a different viral threat: an infodemic.

Spreading as fast as coronavirus is the misinformation about it. Accuracy of information is important to allay fears, subdue panic and to control populations from doing the opposite of what is necessary such as not wearing masks. A search by the New York Times revealed cracks in the monitoring systems. There are cases of hackers creating digital traps aimed at stealing personal data by breaking into devices, false and malicious content triggering conspiracy theories and finger pointing governments for withholding information. The trajectory of fallacies was as profound as the coronavirus bypassing media watchdogs and gatekeepers.

And this is where imagination in forward thinking is necessary.

Both Bill Gates and Larry Brilliant, the latter being the doctor who helped defeat smallpox, explained in 2015 and 1996 respectively, that a looming pandemic was inevitable. While Gates was concerned about the strength of our medical infrastructure to support a pandemic of epic proportions, Brilliant was perturbed by the possible numbers. 'A billion people would get sick,' he said. 'As many as 165 million people would die. There would be a global recession and depression, and the cost to our economy of $1 to $3 trillion would be far worse for everyone than merely 100 million people dying, because so many more people would lose their jobs and their healthcare benefits, that the consequences are almost unthinkable.' Being a scientist, Brilliant projected a worse case scenario to imagine but history has several good examples namely the Spanish flu of 1918 as our cautionary tale. Unfortunately that is not what people are tuned in to. Cradled in their misery, people are seeking comfort in memes and comfort food recipes.

While governments are seeking ways to tape financial leakages, scientists like Brilliant, who is currently chairman of the board of Ending Pandemics, are in a race against time to find a vaccine and get to the 'epidemiologist gold ring'. In his words, 'That means A, a large enough quantity of us have caught the disease and become immune. And B, we have a vaccine. The combination of A plus B is enough to create herd immunity, which is around 70 or 80 per cent.'

Flattening the curve does not mean we eradicate the virus but we can postpone the infection to give us time to get to the vaccine. The reason why it is called novel coronavirus is because it is new. That there is no human being in the world that has immunity as a result of having had it before. That means it's capable of infecting 7.8 billion people and why it is so voracious in nature. Perhaps *that* would have been useful information for the Minister of Health to placate the people rather than act out how to stay hydrated. Within an hour of his segment, the minister has lost the respect of an entire nation, the respect of both the public health community and the political community.

Lesson to be learned here: logistics alone will, over time, desensitize people, but truth and transparency will profound the significance of what is truly happening around a scared nation. And for the public to panic and to feel such, leaders and rulers need to remember, those are valid and powerful human emotions that should not be dumbed down.

Frantic Sketch

It's May 2020.

Announcements have been made about all festive activities being halted for the year. Bollocks.

If we are lucky, the government officials said we can celebrate Christmas. Borders are closed and infection rate increases rapidly. New Year is now wishful thinking.

Turning to my balcony, I do what gives me most comfort, exercise and breathe into the open skies. But in my mind the thoughts keep racing based on all the readings circulating in the media:

The data is coming in
Tons of hypothesis, give the virus time, let the virus rise up and study it.
Lack of consistency.
Why are we responding this way now?
Data was theoretical. Coronavirus has been studied for decades.
Every year there is a new coronavirus. Increase or decrease virulent.
Studies since the seventies.
It sparks fear when a new strain emerges. Risk limitation. Mitigation.
Strategic plan.
A race for vaccines begins.
A race against time.

My brain makes voracious mental notes on its own in its defence of isolation.

Every day you're learning. Look at trends. In 6-8 weeks we have crippled the economy, domestic abuse has increased; is social isolation what is needed at this point? Academics and reality are two different things. Understand the progression of the disease. Fomites.

You listen to the people around you. Everyone becomes a social critic, a virus expert and increasingly depressed. Every day you read stories reeked of fear, sickness and death. Yet, it was reading that held me together.

> *Fomites are being transferred. A total shutdown. Microbiology and immunology.*
> *Our response is wrong.*
> *Testing gives you a moment in time.*
> *Comorbidities.*
> *COVID is part of it. Not a COVID death. Compromised.*
> *COVID has to be added to the Diagnostic list when there is nothing to do with COVID.*
> *Asymptomatic 25 per cent*
> *Widespread*
> *Herd immunity or burns itself out—how a virus dies*
> *It would be safer to be outside without masks.*
> *Building blocks of the immune system are viruses and bacteria.*
> *Opportunistic infection.*

I don't know how Anne Frank survived being locked in the narrow annex. I have more liberty for space yet my mind seems to be crushing upon my sanity while facing a panoramic view at my balcony. Perhaps COVID is as much a mental attack as it is to the respiratory and immune system.

Cognition in crisis

Fighting what we cannot understand is to cut running water with a sword.
Get a grip, Natasha. They say journaling saves nine.
How are the leaders feeling today?

I was reading an article by Prof Neal Ashkanasy from the University of Queensland, Australia titled *More than a feeling: why emotional intelligence is crucial for leaders during a crisis* where he writes: 'The global COVID-19 pandemic has brought about a series of changes to the way we work. From suddenly managing teams working remotely to employees experiencing mental health or financial hardship—the crisis has led to many new leadership challenges.'

In the news, citizens were beginning to observe, comment and criticize the ways leaders were placating nations with the lockdown. Mitigations, tactics and strategies. Suddenly the whole world was a stage. Each premier was a contestant on How to be an Effective Leader. And oh boy, were there many Simon Cowells offering unsolicited points of view on social media. Soon what started as social commentary on leadership became a political critique on gender study. 'The evidence shows a strong correlation between the quality of national leadership and the severity of the pandemic,' says Ashkanasy, who is also helping develop leaders in emotional intelligence through the pandemic as a lecturer into the UQ Master of Business Administration (MBA) program.

Ashkanasy highlights New Zealand Prime Minister Jacinda Ardern as an example of a leader who demonstrates emotional intelligence in her role, particularly during a crisis. 'The way Prime Minister Ardern interacts with people, listens to other points of view, pays attention to what other people say and tries to empathise with them are all signs of emotional intelligence.'

In the business world, Ashkanasy suggests that Qantas CEO Alan Joyce is another prominent leader who has demonstrated this skillset under dire circumstances. 'The way he communicated and explained to staff and customers the horrendous cuts that had to be made for the airline to survive enabled him to successfully steer the fine line between making very difficult business decisions and keeping staff and customers onside.'

Indeed this was a testing time for everyone. Politicians and ministers worth their salt would milk this opportunity to be the heroes of the people. And because people are stuck in their homes, the advantage is that leaders' voices are louder than usual. People needed comforting and assurance on three key areas: moratoriums, vaccines, and lockdowns. People needed support on another three: businesses, mental health, and connection. Information was key yet confusion was often played. Ashkanasy asserts, 'Leadership is an emotion-laden process at the best of times. Under high-stress conditions, like navigating a pandemic, it's more difficult to access our cognitive resources. Leaders who can manage their own emotions, have empathy for others and prioritise relationship-building are most effective in these situations.'

And then this headline went viral on Malaysian social media: '*Talk like Doraemon': Malaysian ministry issues tips for wives during COVID-19 movement control order.*

I choked on my coffee.

As reported on *Channel News Asia*:

Married women in Malaysia were briefly issued a set of recommendations on how to manage their households and husbands during the movement control order, including speaking in 'Doraemon's voice' and giggling coyly.

The Women and Family Ministry on Monday (Mar 30) posted several tips on social media on how to avoid domestic arguments between husband and wife.

The posts, made public on both Facebook and Instagram, were taken down a day later.

'If you see your husband carry out a task in a manner that clashes with your own method, avoid nagging,' the ministry said in a since-deleted infographic.

In a separate image, the ministry said wives should instead use 'humorous' words and phrases such as 'this is the proper way to hang the clothes for drying, my dear (cara sidai baju macam ni lah sayangku)'.

The ministry also recommended that women should 'mimic the tone of Doraemon' and follow their statements with a coy and feminine laugh.

I cringed and sat beside myself in shame I never knew existed. To what madness is this? And an entire ministry? Even Fujiko Fujio would disagree. If this was leadership in my own backyard during an unprecedented crisis at room temperature, I fear what awaits at boiling point. Is this empathy? Is this supposed to be educated advice? Erasmus, the great Renaissance thinker, reminds us, 'The best hope of a nation lies in the proper education of its youth.' What would the younger generation make of this?

COVID-19 has reared an ugly head. Turns out the virus has an insidious sense of humour for bringing out the best and the worst leaders. Sadly, the worst included one of my country's thought leaders for women and family.

I hope Arden isn't scrolling.

Corona: The language, the mist,
the monster

'Flattening the curve does not mean we eradicate the virus but we can postpone the infection to give us time to get to the vaccine. The reason why it is called Novel Coronavirus is because it is new. That there is no human being in the world that has immunity as a result of having had it before. That means it's capable of infecting 7.8 billion people and why it is so voracious in nature.' Larry Brilliant in an interview with Wired.com

In 1980, Stephen King wrote a novella titled *The Mist*. Described as an American science-fiction horror, it became a film in 2007 written and directed by Frank Darabont.

Although a monster movie, the plot revolves around members of the small town of Bridgton, Maine, who after a severe thunderstorm causes the power to go out the night before, meet in a supermarket to pick up supplies. An unnatural mist envelopes the town and to their horror, conceals a vicious entity that seems hell-bent on claiming every life in its path.

The enemy is unclear although for the purpose of Hollywood tropes hints of alien-like monsters are presented. But what exactly it is, we don't know. It is the perfect Lovecraftian horror (also known as cosmic horror) where the fear and awe we feel when confronted by phenomena is beyond our comprehension, whose scope extends beyond the narrow field of human affairs and boasts of cosmic significance.

Signature of King's stories, the central theme explores what ordinary people are driven to do under extraordinary circumstances. Darabont's version focuses on the survivors trapped in the supermarket. Strangers, limitations and lack of trust. Instinct is to flight but they're trapped, forced to fight. As they struggle to survive, extreme tension mounts, and the truth of their humanity surfaces. Selfishness, self-entitlement and fear-induced desperation. There are monsters outside, and there are also monsters inside. Classic Stephen King.

The ending however is the kicker that will haunt you for days.

The protagonist escapes with four other survivors in a vehicle, one being a child. Surrounded by the inescapable deadly mist, the survivors look at each other in despondence, apathy and utter despair. There is no way they can escape what's greater than themselves. The protagonist holds a gun, but there are only four bullets. Not wanting to succumb to the savagery of the mist, they surrender to mercy killing. After shooting them, the protagonist screams in guilt. Now alone in the vehicle with four dead bodies and shrouded by the thickening mist, he opens the door to surrender to the cosmic enemy. Taunting it, he hears a distant rumble approaching. The end is near. Ready to surrender to its brutality, an army tank emerges from the mist with heavily armed soldiers. Another vehicle passes loaded with survivors followed by foot soldiers and hovering military rescue helicopters. There is a moment of suspended belief and incredulity. The protagonist, pained and disconsolate despite seeing the rescue efforts, falls to the ground. The scene ends with his piercing cries of agony.

He realizes that he could've saved them all if he waited just a little longer.

He is rescued. Is he? Killing the others though out of mercy, made him no less a monster than the mist. And while the mist, being the mysterious beast it was, chose to kill indiscriminately, our protagonist realizes it was more vile when you didn't. He had pulled the trigger on people he knew were righteous, deserving to live, and what humanity needed. The child symbolizes hope and the future. He annihilated all that was good and all that was civilized.

COVID-19 in 2020 brings no mist. There are no claws, no growling, no rumblings in the distance. But we are shrouded by so much data that may be working against us. There are fatalities, there are agents of rescue, and the screams are by citizens frustrated by the inconsistencies of governmental instructions, by broken economic systems, and by not knowing what the future holds. COVID-19 is a pandemic no deadlier than the Spanish flu in 1918 and the Bubonic Plague in the mid-1300s. To date there have been five deadly pandemics: Plague of Justinian, the Black Death, The Great Plague of London, smallpox and cholera. What killed a fraction of the world's population at each blow is the newness of it all. And linguistics.

Bugs don't die, they multiply

'The limits of my language means the limits of my world.'
Ludwig Wittgenstein

The Plague of Justinian arrived in Constantinople, the capital of the Byzantine Empire, in 541 CE. It was carried over the Mediterranean Sea from Egypt, a recently conquered land paying tribute to Emperor Justinian in grain. Plague-ridden fleas hitched a ride on the black rats that snacked on the grain. The plague decimated Constantinople and spread like wildfire across Europe, Asia, North Africa and Arabia killing an estimated 30-50 million people, perhaps half of the world's population.

'People had no real understanding of how to fight it other than trying to avoid sick people,' says Thomas Mockaitis, a history professor at DePaul University. 'As to how the plague ended, the best guess is that the majority of people in a pandemic somehow survive, and those who survive have immunity.'

These plagues never went away. They evolved, assimilated, took different disguises to adapt into our varied ecosystems. And so did we. But with every deadly episode, each left characteristic imprints that help us to make better sense of the world we live in. These imprints were in the form of new strains, new science and new lexicon. And it is the latter we should not take for granted.

Interestingly, the speculation surrounding the origin of COVID-19 is different. A new player. Conspiracy theories range from a lab experiment turned awry, a zoonotic pathogen carried by bats through an ecological disruption, to a bio-engineered warfare intended for global attack. Novel here means we are alien to a collective vocabulary. From rising unemployment statistics to promising drug trials, new information about this pandemic emerges constantly, and dozens of theories about how the disease spreads and can be treated get advanced or disproven on any given day. Our best bet is to compare notes from yesteryears with the hope that there's a match to something experts are familiar with.

And this is where the Sapir-Whorf hypothesis comes in.

What they know shapes what we know

Benjamin Lee Whorf was an American linguist known as an advocate for the idea that because of linguistic differences in grammar and usage, speakers of different languages conceptualize and experience the world differently. He describes, 'We dissect nature along lines laid down by our native language. Language is not simply a reporting device for experience but a defining framework for it.' But most profoundly, 'Language shapes the way we think, and determines what we can think about.'

Edward Sapir, arguably the most influential figure in American linguistics, has this to say about the relation between language, culture and cognition in his book *The Status Of Linguistics as a Science* (1929): 'The worlds in which different societies live are distinct worlds, not merely the same world with different labels attached. We see and hear and otherwise experience very largely as we do because the language habits of our community predispose certain choices of interpretation.'

Both linguists were challenged against the normative belief that language presented cognitive universals of cultural differences. Just as there are stock characters identifiable in literature, there are universal signs and signifiers that allow us to understand one another regardless of where we come from.

Every day since WHO declared COVID-19 a pandemic threat, we have been armed by nothing more than the building blocks of conflicting information pieced together by the worlds' best and brightest's understanding. In short, what they know shapes what we know. And as the saying goes by Desiderius Erasmus, 'In the kingdom of the blind, the one eye is king.' And that in itself should be a terrifying thought. We are surrounded by a mist of uncertainty but seminal in shaping new policies that will govern our future, affect our behaviour and influence global leaders.

According to a COVID-19 report by Wired magazine, 'The 2019 coronavirus is one of hundreds we know of, and one of seven known to infect humans. These viruses affect the lungs and also cause fever and sometimes gastrointestinal problems. The WHO declared the coronavirus situation a global emergency in January and a pandemic in mid-March. The most common symptoms of COVID-19 are dry cough, fever, and shortness of breath. Others include diarrhoea and loss of smell or taste. Some people develop severe blood clots. The disease is mercurial, fairly mild for some and fatal for others. Scientists can't say definitively why, but women are less likely to die than men. We know that older people, especially those with underlying health issues, are more at risk. And children fare better than adults, but for babies, toddlers, and kids with other conditions the disease can be severe.'

Our response: Lockdown, partial lockdown. Quarantine. Restricted movement control orders. Declaration of emergency. Repeated state of emergencies. Mask on. Mask off. Mandatory mask. Social distancing. Riots. Retaliation. Resistance. Global crisis. Work from home (WFH). Race for vaccines. Fear. Anger. Anxiety. The Other.

By textbook definition we know what these words mean. They are now thrusted upon us to create a new framework that underpins our life. They call it the new normal. But what exactly is the new normal?

It is not the expansion of thought but the restriction of knowledge

COVID-19 is a great challenge to us because of its temperamental personality. Nebulous. It has been kinder on regions such as Vietnam, Thailand and New Zealand but brutally harsh in Italy, Spain and the United States. Why is this so? Experts remain baffled by its constitution resulting in conflating reports.

In October 2020 we are experiencing its second wave, or third, or perhaps we've only just graced the onset of its germination. Many countries reissued lockdowns. A second round made people incredibly reactive. Citizens were also losing their patience and trust in governments. Previous summers gave us a slew of Marvel hero movies. Today we feel cheated by Hollywood as in truth there is none. Our mortal heroes wear suits, battle bureaucratic tape and are susceptible to corruption and scandals. Their sworn enemies are those who oppose their political views. Trump versus Biden. Not exactly the poetic justice we seek. No CGI. In September, nine rival pharmaceutical companies, among them Pfizer, BioNTech, Moderna, and AstraZeneca, pledged that any coronavirus vaccine they produce will be developed and tested with 'high ethical standards and sound scientific principles,' in a bid to help ensure public confidence. Standard approval process by the Food and Drug Administration (FDA) typically takes years. With COVID-19, to speed up FDA is willing to issue the emergency authorization which has proven highly controversial. And why wouldn't it be?

While researchers race in laboratories, citizens the world over wait with bated breath for vaccines while working in their bedrooms, kitchens and living rooms. Ten months into 2020 it was citizens who were also fighting wars for democracy.

A Room with a view

Months into the lockdown it was easy to forget what day it was. A routine soon takes place and you forget the calendar has numbers. I wake up, read the news updates, reach out for the mandatory caffeine fix. Many nights I go to bed looking forward to that morning cup of coffee. Algorithms feed you your staple diet. Mine consisted of geopolitics, economics, culture and communication. Perhaps during a pandemic, this is a bad idea. A composite of distress. A close friend who suffers from anxiety often intermittently fasts from reading the news, opting to stare at his blank walls for comfort. I don't blame him. I am, however, a sucker for pain, a glutton for punishment.

As much as possible, I avoid the celebrity gossip and trivial chatter on TikTok, Instagram and Facebook despite the entire village being there. Yes, social media connects you to the world but often I beg the question, *is it a world I want to be connected to?* The content on those platforms are entertaining but they also perturb my anxiety because society often ate itself like an ouroboros: Local celebrities get pregnant with a COVID baby, and suddenly to procreate a COVID baby seems like a great idea while the world screams in agony of overpopulation, pollution and civil unrest. Let's not forget we are *still* being held hostage by a virus that is overwhelming hospitals, reducing mankind and depleting the economy.

The mind needs to sink its teeth into something that can keep the synapses flickering and electricity voltage conducting alternating and direct current. For me, I found solace in the tundra of podcasts and periodicals where reports were high on objectivity and low on sensationalism. My online shopping consisted of subscriptions to the *Economist*, the *New Yorker*, the *Atlantic*, *Reader's Digest*, *Bloomberg* and

Forbes Asia. In that sense I had it better than Anne Frank. I had IoT, the Internet of Things.

It was through this edited window that I became more aware of a world in chaos. Its dark web. The pre-pandemic world, it seems, was already a mess. COVID-19 added more salt. I saw connections from one continent to another, patterns of Governmentality and the polarisation of social injustice brought upon by religion, social classes and corruption. Previously, the dailiness of our routined life distracted us from what was happening in the larger social spheres. Lockdown and IoT creates and amplifies parasocial interaction.

What I found intriguing was the interpolated narratives woven in those socio-economic gaps. Many things didn't add up. Mostly because they had tentacles from the past. Henry Kissinger wrote, 'It is not often that nations learn from the past, even rarer that they draw the correct conclusions from it.' COVID-19 was a malefactor revealing pain points in the way we managed modern life, some I knew existed, some I didn't realize were in dire straits. Reading in COVID captivity, I realized Kissinger didn't write books. He wrote oracles. In *World Order: Reflections on the Character of Nations and the Course of History,* Kissinger describes eloquently the modus operandi of many leaders handling the COVID crisis:

> Because information is so accessible and communication instantaneous, there is a diminution of focus on its significance, or even on the definition of what is significant. This dynamic may encourage policymakers to wait for an issue to arise rather than anticipate it, and to regard moments of decision as a series of isolated events rather than part of a historical continuum. When this happens, manipulation of information replaces reflection as the principal policy tool.

Steal the milk, rape the cow

It was a slow October crawling into November.

High on my observation list was an uptick on totalitarianism and authoritarianism while human rights and democracy were slipping.

COVID articles for the week:

India fights a battle against insufficient testing with 7.9 million people infected and 120,000 deaths. Among the countries worst affected by COVID, India's biggest problem is infrastructure to expedite testing. According to the WHO report, there is an estimate of 1,126 government and 883 laboratories, many districts have only one laboratory. Majority of the laboratories are in the 36 state and union territories' capital cities. India's communities depend largely on community-based monitoring (CBM), a form of public oversight, aimed to generate the appropriate information to seek and strengthen local decision-making, public education, community capacity and effective public participation in local government. But there was a more consequential problem added to the battle. Rural areas, compared to the urban, had very limited digital access creating a social dissonance regarding information and urgency for testing.

Indonesia scrambles between saving lives and its economy leading President Joko Widodo to approve a dubious 'omnibus' law provoking riots. Widodo championed a law which cuts red tape to stimulate investment but at the expense of weakening protection for workers and the environment. The law reduces the autonomy enjoyed by provincial, district and city governments across the archipelago as well as the say of affected communities in the issuing of environmental permits. The law will create a significant chain of events: it removes royalties, lowers tax, eases logging and encourages deforestation.

In Thailand where COVID-19 has spared kindness (3,759 infected, fatality rate of 59 as of October 27), students and activists have directed their protests squarely at the monarchy, an institution previously held as sacred. The Thai monarchy is fiercely guarded by a draconian law punishable by years in prison for the slightest criticism, a law known as Lèse-majesté. Since the October 2016 death of Bhumibol, Thailand's new King, Maha Vajiralongkorn has moved to consolidate political power and assume control over billions of dollars of assets from the Crown Property Bureau and the command of the 1st and 11th Infantry Regiments, based in Bangkok. The King has taken stakes in major Thai companies such as Siam Commercial Bank and Siam Cement, as well as vast amounts of land. Rather than build his own legacy, Vajiralongkorn has used the legitimacy gained by his father over decades to bend the military to his will. Many top-ranking officers, like Royal Thai Army Chief General Apirat Kongsompong, were hand-picked by Vajiralongkorn himself. All these by spending considerable time in Germany half-naked in small, tight top crops surrounded by women in a self-imposed Bavarian luxury hotel courtesy of the 70 million Thais located 5,000 miles away.

The Malaysian government headed by prime minister Muhyiddin Yassin decides to use COVID-19 to a different advantage—to abuse the Malaysian federal constitution to suspend parliament to approve its 2021 budget without parliamentary approval. The audacity in wanting to declare an emergency citing COVID-19 against dubious data (out of 28,640 infected cases, 238 deaths reported as of 28 October) shows contempt for the rule of law and the basic principles of constitutional government.

Despite many countries issuing partial to total lockdowns Russia's Vladimir Putin refuses to give in to the virus. On October 16, infections have proliferated with 15,700 new cases. By October 21 its health care system was looking at 1,447,335 infections in total. The country of around 145 million people has the world's fourth largest caseload after the United States, India and Brazil. But Putin remains adamant to avoid a lockdown. 'Russia is not planning to impose any blanket restrictions to contain the COVID-19 pandemic.' He added, 'Regarding the possibility of harsh, total measures—we are not planning to do it. The government does not have such plans,' Putin said at a meeting held by video link with Russia's top business figures.

We are barely seven months into the pandemic.

We are uncertain of the future and every day we are learning about COVID-19 and its behaviour. The same can be said about people. We are restricted by action due to our limited understanding. Yet, governments, leaders and influential figures are advancing in various strategies to milk what they can from this pandemic.

Are we back in the mist?

The girl who cried whorf

The Sapir-Whorf hypothesis posits that the structure of language greatly influences the models of thought and behaviour characteristic to the culture in which it is spoken.

After his extensive study on Mesoamerican linguistics, Whorf was a believer that language carried layers of meaning and interpretation. With COVID-19 we are presented with various interpretations of the virus depending on how advanced your laboratory is, how much funding you're supported, and by which government. Current methodology to understand how it spreads and mutates is through a wait-and-watch approach. In between these uncertainties, governments weigh up the trade-offs of each restriction such as whether or not to close schools, to enforce a mask mandate or to adhere to a full or partial lockdown. Governments like China take the authoritative approach while others like Sweden are more liberty-loving. Several countries like Taiwan and South Korea have clear, consistent messages on rapid large-scale testing to identify and suppress outbreaks early, while others like Indonesia are lax on contact tracing and the United Kingdom and United States delayed calls for action. Unavoidable casualties include schools forced to shut down, increase in unemployment, distributed organizations, and micro, small to medium enterprises shutting down.

But should this be new to us? Shouldn't we have a common language to defeat pandemics by now? What have we learned and not learned? Is it due to lack of documentation or because of complacency that we remain divisive on tackling COVID-19?

In the case of the plague in 1347, it never really went away, and when it returned 800 years later, it killed with reckless abandon. The

Black Death, which hit predominantly Europe, claimed 200 million lives in four years. According to historians the plague resurfaced roughly every ten years from 1348 to 1665: forty outbreaks in over 300 years.

'As for how to stop the disease, people still had no scientific understanding of contagion,' says Thomas Mockaitis, a history professor at DePaul University, but they knew that it had something to do with proximity. 'That's why forward-thinking officials in Venetian-controlled port city of Ragusa decided to keep newly arrived sailors in isolation until they could prove they weren't sick. At first, sailors were held on their ships for thirty days, which became known in Venetian law as a *trentino*. As time went on, the Venetians increased the forced isolation to forty days or a *quarantino*, the origin of the word quarantine and the start of its practice in the Western world.'

So is the COVID-19 really that novel of a virus? And if outbreaks have been resurfacing since the Middle Ages, why do we act incipiently?

Feels like Bill Murray's groundhog day

The earliest recorded pandemic happened in Athens during the Peloponnesian War in 430 BC. After the disease passed through Libya, Ethiopia and Egypt, it crossed the Athenian walls as the Spartans laid siege. As much as two-thirds of the population died. The symptoms included fever, thirst, bloody throat and tongue, red skin and lesions. The disease, suspected to have been typhoid fever, weakened the Athenians significantly and was a critical factor in their defeat by the Spartans.

In the eleventh century, leprosy grew into a pandemic in Europe resulting in the building of numerous leprosy-focused hospitals to accommodate the vast number of victims. A slow-developing bacterial disease that causes sores and deformities, leprosy was believed to be a punishment from God that ran in families. This belief led to moral judgments and ostracization of victims. Now known as Hansen's disease, it still afflicts tens of thousands of people a year and can be fatal if not treated with antibiotics.

In 1492, upon arrival on the island of Hispaniola, Christopher Columbus encountered the Taino people, population 60,000. By 1548, the population stood at less than 500. This scenario repeated itself throughout the Americas. In 1520, the Aztec Empire was destroyed by a smallpox infection. The disease killed many of its victims and incapacitated others. It weakened the population so they were unable to resist Spanish colonizers and left farmers unable to produce needed crops. Research in 2019 even concluded that the deaths of some fifty-six million Native Americans in the sixteenth and seventeenth centuries, largely through disease, may have altered Earth's climate as vegetation growth on previously tilled land drew more CO2 from the atmosphere and caused a cooling event.

As cholera tore through England, killing tens of thousands within days of the first symptoms, a British doctor named John Snow suspected that the mysterious disease lurked in London's drinking water. Prevailing scientific theory of the day said that the disease was spread by foul air known as a miasma. Investigating hospital records and morgue reports to track the precise locations of deadly outbreaks, Snow created a geographic chart of cholera deaths over a ten-day period, and found a cluster of 500 fatal infections surrounding the Broad Street pump, a popular city well for drinking water. Snow convinced local officials to remove the pump handle on the Broad Street drinking well, rendering it unusable, and the infections dried up. Snow's work didn't cure cholera overnight, but it improved urban sanitation and protected drinking water from contamination.

With every epoch of disaster, mankind learned to redefine and better acquaint with his environment. With reference to the Sapir-Whorf hypothesis, it developed our vocabulary in connection with culture and society improving marvel science through medicine, healthcare, social welfare, architecture, economics, agriculture and aspects of public policies. At least that's ideally how it *should* be.

Increasing literature on vaccines

'Everyone had a fear there would be explosive outbreaks of [coronavirus] transmission in the schools. In colleges, there have been. We have to say that, to date, we have not seen those in the younger kids, and that is a really important observation.'
Michael Osterholm, Washington Post, 23 September 2020

Before citizens can cry foul or protest the delay in finding 'the cure', rigorous understanding is required to break down the science of the virus. Achieving this is not only expensive but requires a collective effort by many experts at every level. Scientists the world over are parsing goals into smaller, manageable, and realistic parts. The cross-collaboration is critical to assist policy makers understand how new technologies could improve healthcare, and the actions needed to put innovations into practice. Osterholm adds, 'The public health community wants a safe and effective [COVID-19] vaccine as much as anybody could want it. But the data have to be clear and compelling.'

According to the University of Cambridge, coronavirus SARS-CoV-2, the virus behind the COVID-19 pandemic, has been studied intensely since emerging in late 2019 — so far, researchers have sequenced tens of thousands of SARS-CoV-2 genomes to learn about the genetic variation of the virus. Monitoring the viral genome for mutations can give important clues as to how the biology of the virus is changing and the potential impact on transmission rates and disease severity. From a policy point of view, this can have huge impacts on reinstating or relaxing lockdown and social distancing measures.

Based on the *New York Times*, as early as January 2020 scientists have been deciphering the SARS-CoV-2 genome triggered by the alarms of the Wuhan outbreak.

The first vaccine safety trials in humans started in March, and as of October, ten have reached the final stages of testing. Researchers are testing forty-eight vaccines in clinical trials on humans, and at least eighty-eight preclinical vaccines are under active investigation in animals. There are five stages to this process. The following is an excerpt from the *New York Times* Coronavirus Vaccine Tracker:

PRECLINICAL TESTING: Scientists test a new vaccine on cells and then give it to animals such as mice or monkeys to see if it produces an immune response. We have confirmed 88 preclinical vaccines in active development.

PHASE 1 SAFETY TRIALS: Scientists give the vaccine to a small number of people to test safety and dosage as well as to confirm that it stimulates the immune system.

PHASE 2 EXPANDED TRIALS: Scientists give the vaccine to hundreds of people split into groups, such as children and the elderly, to see if the vaccine acts differently in them. These trials further test the vaccine's safety and ability to stimulate the immune system.

PHASE 3 EFFICACY TRIALS: Scientists give the vaccine to thousands of people and wait to see how many become infected, compared with volunteers who received a placebo. These trials can determine if the vaccine protects against the coronavirus. In June, the F.D.A. advised vaccine makers that they would want to see evidence that vaccines can protect at least 50 percent of those who receive it. In addition, Phase 3 trials are large enough to reveal evidence of relatively rare side effects that might be missed in earlier studies.

EARLY OR LIMITED APPROVAL: China and Russia have approved vaccines without waiting for the results of Phase 3 trials. Experts say the rushed process has serious risks.

APPROVAL: Regulators in each country review the trial results and decide whether to approve the vaccine or not. During a pandemic, a vaccine may receive emergency use authorization before getting formal approval. Once a vaccine is licensed, researchers continue to monitor people who receive it to make sure it's safe and effective.

Additional note: **COMBINED PHASES:** One way to accelerate vaccine development is to combine phases. Some coronavirus vaccines are now in Phase 1/2 trials, for example, in which they are tested for the first time on hundreds of people. (Note that our tracker counts a combined Phase 1/2 trial as both Phase 1 and Phase 2)

PAUSED: If investigators observe worrying symptoms in volunteers, they can put a trial on pause. After an investigation, the trial may resume or be abandoned.

But then there is also the issue of trust. Michael Osterholm, an American epidemiologist, regents professor, and director of the Centre for Infectious Disease Research and Policy at the University of Minnesota has been vocal at every step of the process.

> There is a pattern here that has occurred over a number of topics for both agencies [FDA and CDC] over the period of recent weeks that is making a lot of people in the public health community at state and local and federal levels doubt the scientific integrity of these agencies—which is the worst thing that we can have happen to us in terms of public health credibility.
> *Stat News*, 27 August 2020

In *Voice of America* on 5 August 2020 he said, 'Will we have a COVID-19 vaccine or vaccines by the end of the year? Likely.

But the question is, what does that mean? Will it be rushed in terms of its evaluation such that people lack confidence in it? How long will it protect for, even if it is adequately evaluated and the safety issues around it elucidated? We just don't know that yet.'

Back to the Sapir-Whorf hypothesis: We can only advance as far as we know based on knowledge that is grounded in supporting scientific evidence. And so we turn to the scientific evidence we can confirm:

Genetic vaccines. These are vaccines that deliver one or more of the coronavirus's own genes into our cells to provoke an immune response. These are vaccines based on messenger RNA (mRNA) to produce viral proteins in the body. RNA based vaccines could have an impact in these areas due to their shorter manufacturing times and greater effectiveness.

Unlike a normal vaccine, RNA vaccines work by introducing an mRNA sequence (the molecule which tells cells what to build) which is coded for a disease specific antigen, once produced within the body, the antigen is recognised by the immune system, preparing it to fight the real thing. RNA vaccines are faster and cheaper to produce than traditional vaccines, and a RNA based vaccine is also safer for the patient, as they are not produced using infectious elements. Production of RNA vaccines is laboratory based, and the process could be standardised and scaled, allowing quick responses to large outbreaks and epidemics.

As reported by *NYT*,

The German company BioNTech entered into collaborations with Pfizer, based in New York, and the Chinese drug maker Fosun Pharma to develop an mRNA vaccine to be given in two doses. In May they launched a Phase 1/2 trial on two versions of the vaccine. They found that both versions caused volunteers to produce antibodies against SARS-CoV-2, as well as immune cells called T cells that respond to the virus. They found that one version, called BNT162b2, produced significantly fewer side effects, such as fevers and fatigue, and so they chose it to move into Phase 2/3 trials. On July 27, the companies announced the launch of a Phase 2/3 trial with 30,000 volunteers in the United States and other countries including Argentina, Brazil, and Germany. In an interim study, the companies reported that after getting the first dose, volunteers experience mostly mild to moderate side effects. On Sept. 12, Pfizer and BioNTech announced that they would seek to expand their U.S. trial to 43,000 participants. The following month, they gained permission to start testing the vaccine on children as young as 12—the first American trial to do so.

In September, Dr Albert Bourla, the chief executive of Pfizer, said the Phase 3 trial would deliver enough results as soon as October to show if the vaccine worked or not. On Oct. 27, Dr Bourla announced that the volunteers in the trial had yet to experience enough cases of COVID-19 to determine if the vaccines work.

Pfizer and BioNTech's vaccine, like almost all the others in clinical trials, requires two doses. In the summer, the companies began inking deals to deliver large orders to countries around the world. The Trump administration awarded a $1.9 billion contract in July for 100 million doses to be delivered by December and the option to acquire 500 million more doses. Meanwhile, Japan made a deal for 120 million doses, and the European Union arranged to purchase 200 million doses. If their vaccine is authorized, Pfizer and BioNTech expect to manufacture over 1.3 billion doses of their vaccine worldwide by the end of 2021.

Getting the vaccine from the factory to people's arms could pose some major challenges. Pfizer and BioNTech preparation is based on mRNA, which falls apart unless it's kept in a deep freeze. As a result, the vaccine will have to be chilled to minus 80 degrees Celsius (minus 112 degrees Fahrenheit) until it's ready to be injected.

In October, South Korea faced a public panic sparked by news headlines in September fifty-nine people died after receiving flu shots. Some headline also mentioned that 480,000 doses of flu vaccines were momentarily exposed to room temperature. This lead to President Moon Jae-in to urge South Koreans to trust health authorities.

The vaccines were all recalled but this lapse heightened distrust in COVID-19 vaccines.

Viral vector vaccines. These are vaccines that contain viruses engineered to carry coronavirus genes. Some viral vector vaccines enter cells and cause them to make viral proteins. Other viral vectors slowly replicate, carrying coronavirus proteins on their surface.

As reported by *NYT*,

> The Gamaleya Research Institute, part of Russia's Ministry of Health, launched clinical trials in June of a vaccine they called Gam-COVID-Vac. It is a combination of two adenoviruses, Ad5 and Ad26, both engineered with a coronavirus gene.
>
> On Aug. 11, President Vladimir V. Putin announced that a Russian health care regulator had approved the vaccine, renamed Sputnik V, before Phase 3 trials had even begun. Vaccine experts decried the move as risky, and Russia later walked back the announcement, saying that the approval was a 'conditional registration certificate,' which would depend on positive results from Phase 3 trials. Those trials, initially planned for just 2,000 volunteers, were expanded to 40,000. In addition to Russia, volunteers were recruited in Belarus, the United Arab Emirates, and Venezuela. On Oct. 17, a Phase 2/3 trial was launched in India.
>
> On Sept. 4, three weeks after Putin's announcement, Gamaleya researchers published the results of their Phase 1/2 trial. In a small study, they found that Sputnik yielded antibodies to the coronavirus and mild side effects. Meanwhile, Russia negotiated agreements to supply the vaccine to countries including Brazil, Mexico and India.

Protein-based vaccines. Vaccines that contain coronavirus proteins but no genetic material. Some vaccines contain whole proteins, and some contain fragments of them. Some pack many of these molecules on nanoparticles.

As reported by *NYT*,

Maryland-based Novavax makes vaccines by sticking proteins onto microscopic particles. They've taken on a number of different diseases this way; their flu vaccine finished Phase 3 trials in March. The company launched trials for a COVID-19 vaccine in May, and the Coalition for Epidemic Preparedness Innovations has invested $384 million in the vaccine. In July the U.S. government awarded $1.6 billion to support the vaccine's clinical trials and manufacturing.

After getting promising results from preliminary studies in monkeys and humans, Novavax launched a Phase 2 trial in South Africa in August. The blinded, placebo-controlled trial on 2,900 people will measure not just the safety of the vaccine but its efficacy. The following month, Novavax launched a Phase 3 trial enrolling up to 10,000 volunteers in the United Kingdom. It could potentially deliver results by the start of 2021. A larger Phase 3 trial is in development to launch in the United States in October.

If the trials succeed, Novavax expects to deliver 100 million doses for use in the United States by the first quarter of 2021. In September Novavax reached an agreement with the Serum Institute of India, a major vaccine manufacturer, that they said would enable them to produce as many as 2 billion doses a year.

Inactivated or Attenuated Coronavirus Vaccines. These are vaccines created from weakened coronaviruses or coronaviruses that have been killed with chemicals. As of September 15, NYT reports:

The Wuhan Institute of Biological Products developed an inactivated virus vaccine, which the state-owned Chinese company Sinopharm put into clinical tests. The Phase 1/2 trial showed that the vaccine produced antibodies in volunteers, some of whom experienced fevers and other side effects. They launched Phase 3 trials in the United Arab Emirates in July, and in Peru and Morocco the following month. Over the summer, the company later said, the government gave it approval to inject hundreds of thousands of people with its two experimental vaccines. On Sept. 14, the U.A.E. gave emergency approval for Sinopharm's vaccine to use on health care workers.

Sinopharm also began testing a second inactivated virus vaccine, this one developed by the Beijing Institute of Biological Products. After running early clinical trials in China, they launched Phase 3 trials in the United Arab Emirates and Argentina. Over the summer, the company later said, the government gave it approval to inject hundreds of thousands of people with its two experimental vaccines. On Sept. 14, the U.A.E. gave emergency approval for Sinopharm's vaccine to use on health care workers before Sinopharm shared data indicating it was safe and effective. In October, the chairman of Sinopharm said the company was gearing up manufacturing for their two vaccines, with plans for producing a billion doses a year.

Repurposed Vaccines. Vaccines already in use for other diseases that may also protect against COVID-19. Repurposed vaccines are not included in our vaccine count. An example is the Bacillus Calmette-Guerin vaccine. Developed in the early 1900s as a protection against tuberculosis, the Murdoch Children's Research Institute in Australia is conducting a Phase 3 trial called the BRACE to see if the vaccine partly protects against the coronavirus.

This is a disease (COVID-19) that we will be studying for decades and decades to come, just by the very nature of its unique presentations, all the different organs it affected, how it impacted on our immune systems and what then happened because of the dysfunction of our immune systems brought on by this virus. Osterholm, *CBS News Radio*, 22 July 2020

Larry Brilliant, an American epidemiologist, technologist, philanthropist, and author, notable for his 1973-1976 work with the World Health Organization helping to successfully eradicate smallpox, has this to say in March 2020: 'I hold out hope that we get an antiviral for COVID-19 that is curative, but in addition is prophylactic. It's certainly unproven and it's certainly controversial, and certainly a lot of people are not going to agree with me.' Brilliant was referring to two studies published in 2005 in Nature and Science. One of the researchers, Neil Ferguson from Imperial College London, UK, reports:

> If Asian bird flu mutates into a form that spreads easily between humans, an outbreak of just 40 infected people would be enough to cause a global pandemic. And within a year half of the world's population would be infected with a mortality rate of 50 per cent, according to two studies released on Wednesday. And yet, the models show, if targeted action is taken within a critical three-week window, an outbreak could be limited to fewer than 100 individuals within two months.

But, the researchers caution, we are currently far from ready to take the necessary action.

Ferguson further explains in an article for *New Scientist*: 'It represents the first opportunity in history to make use of new knowledge and logistics to prevent a pandemic whose potential loss of life could dwarf the horrific 1918 influenza pandemic. An outbreak is no longer an "if" scenario, it's about "when".'

Ferguson's study in Nature, modelled the potential spread of a bird flu (H5N1) outbreak throughout Thailand's 85 million people. Ira Longini's study, published in *Science*, focused on the nation's 500,000-strong Nang Rong region.

The following is an excerpt taken from *New Scientist* by Gaia Vince titled 'Flu Pandemic, Lethal Yet Preventable':

> The two studies modelled hundreds of scenarios, looking at how the virus could spread person-to-person through different modes of contact, and the effect of various methods of mitigation. For example, simulations were run to model the effects of prophylactic treatment, quarantine, as well as investigating the impact of differing strains and different rates of detection.
>
> The key findings of both studies were in agreement: in order for a nascent pandemic to be controlled there needs to be 3 million courses of oseltamivir (Tamiflu)—the antiviral drug— available for the World Health Organization to mobilise and

deploy internationally, immediately. There also needs to be good surveillance systems in place at the local level, particularly in at-risk countries in south-east Asia, for fast detection of the virus's emergence and accurate diagnosis.

The WHO has stockpiled 120,000 courses of the antiviral drug, far too small a supply to halt an outbreak, the studies warn. The virus needs to be detected within 21 days and before 40 people contract it, the researchers say. Accurate medical diagnosis based on symptoms is key, since by the time results from genetic tests arrive, it will almost certainly be too late. In rural communities with poorly coordinated healthcare provision, swift detection and isolation of cluster groups could prove limited, they add. Likewise, where countries are not immediately open – allowing international intervention in an outbreak – the consequences could be dire. This was what happened during China's SARS virus outbreak.

Following diagnosis of a cluster of infected individuals, the next and hardest task is to prevent the disease spreading, Ferguson says. This should be done through social distancing methods, such as closing schools, travel restrictions and even quarantine. Each new case must be isolated and treated within two days. Populations in a radius surrounding the cluster should be treated with antivirals.

This was in 2005.

According to the Centres for Disease Control and Prevention (CDC) since 1918, the world has experienced three additional pandemics, in 1957, 1968, and 2009. These subsequent pandemics were less severe and caused considerably lower mortality rates than the 1918 pandemic. The 1957 H2N2 pandemic and the 1968 H3N2 pandemic each resulted in an estimated one million global deaths, while the 2009 H1N1 pandemic resulted in fewer than 0.3 million deaths in its first year. One virus in particular has garnered international attention and concern: the avian influenza A(H7N9) virus from China. The H7N9 virus has so far caused 1,568 human infections in China with a case-fatality proportion of about 39 per cent since 2013. However, it has not gained the capability to spread quickly and efficiently between people.

CDC admits while reflecting on the considerable medical, scientific and societal advancements that have occurred since 1918, there are gaps for improvement to prepare us for the next pandemic outbreak. And the list is not short.

CDC attests that the federal government had no centralized role in helping to plan or initiate these interventions during the 1918 pandemic. Mitigation measures included closing schools, banning public gatherings, and issuing isolation or quarantine orders.

Sounds familiar. How much have we improved since 1918?

The world population has grown to 7.8 billion people in 2020. The world population is projected to reach 9.9 billion by 2050. As human populations increase so does the number of hosts. This provides increased opportunities for novel influenza viruses from birds and pigs to spread, evolve and infect people. WHO's Global Influenza Surveillance and Response System (GISRS) is a global flu surveillance network that monitors changes in seasonal flu viruses and also monitors the emergence of novel flu viruses, many of which originate from animal populations.

Challenges at a global level include surveillance capacity, infrastructure and pandemic planning. The majority of countries that report to the WHO still do not have a national pandemic plan, and critical and clinical care capacity, especially in low income countries, continues to be inadequate to the demands of a severe pandemic.

In 2005, milestones were created in the revised International Health Regulations (IHR) for countries to improve their response capacity for public health emergencies, but in 2016, only one-third of countries were in compliance.

If CDC holds the highest level of authority to provide us with knowledge that can protect us from the next pandemic, this is not comforting.

Wrapping my brain around all this information a quote by Frank Sonnenberg comes to mind: 'Lessons in life will be repeated until they are learned.' If we are the architect of our existence and knowledge shapes us, what are we doing with what we do know? Are we deliberately ignoring the signs?

Are we waiting for the mist?

A world on fire

Often it is in the madness of the everyday repetitiveness that I question the rationality of the world. Why is this happening? What are we to learn from all of this? And that is when The Pulley, a poem I learned as a child, would visit me in my COVID afterthought. Perhaps a reminder that one needs to take a break from the media headlines and fear mongering, and to rest in its respite.

The Pulley by George Herbert

When God at first made man,
Having a glass of blessings standing by,
'Let us,' said he, 'pour on him all we can.
Let the world's riches, which dispersèd lie,
Contract into a span.'

So strength first made a way;
Then beauty flowed, then wisdom, honour, pleasure.
When almost all was out, God made a stay,
Perceiving that, alone of all his treasure,
Rest in the bottom lay.

'For if I should,' said he,
'Bestow this jewel also on my creature,
He would adore my gifts instead of me,
And rest in Nature, not the God of Nature;
So both should losers be.

'Yet let him keep the rest,
But keep them with repining restlessness;

Let him be rich and weary, that at least,
If goodness lead him not, yet weariness
May toss him to my breast.'

As we witness global societies retaliate with screams of 'don't tell me what to do', this poem is a balm and a painkiller to remind us that surrendering to what we cannot control is strategic kindness to the overthinking human mind. We need a contention to keep us humble. We need an outbreak to teach us to fix broken systems. The ones that governmental arrogance had allowed swindling and corruption. Perhaps this is timely and this is rightfully what we deserve.

In *Emotional Intelligence: Why It Can Matter More Than IQ*, Goleman writes:

… channelling emotions toward a productive end is a master aptitude. Whether it be in controlling impulse and putting off gratification, regulating our moods so they facilitate rather than impede thinking, motivating ourselves to persist and try, try again in the face of setbacks, or finding ways to enter flow and so perform more effectively—all bespeak the power of emotion to guide effective effort.

Free speech, but at the price of others

'This kindness will I show.
Go with me to a notary, seal me there
Your single bond; and, in a merry sport,
If you repay me not on such a day,
In such a place, such sum or sums as are
Express'd in the condition, let the forfeit
Be nominated for an equal pound
Of your fair flesh, to be cut off and taken
In what part of your body pleaseth me.'

Merchant of Venice by William Shakespeare (1596-1599)

Headlines grew insidious. Unsure if it was the cause or effect of the pandemic frustration. Paris has been on high alert since two journalists from a film production company were stabbed outside the former offices of the satirical newspaper *Charlie Hebdo*. In January 2015, Islamist terrorists Saïd and Chérif Kouachi gunned down twelve people in and around the *Charlie Hebdo* offices. The following day, gunman Amédy Coulibaly shot a policewoman dead and killed four Jewish people at the Hyper Cacher kosher supermarket. The Kouachi brothers and Coulibaly were killed in separate shootouts with police. The trial of fourteen people suspected of being linked to the January 2015 terror attacks is currently being held in a Paris court and is due to continue until November 2020. Ever since, France has been teething with consternation regarding race and religion. Vengeance was always at a tipping point.

On 16 October 2020, forty-seven year old French school teacher Samuel Paty was beheaded by Islamic extremists. His crime? Attempting to teach the concept of 'Liberté, Egalité, Fraternité' using caricatures from *Charlie Hebdo* to a classroom of thirteen year olds. It wasn't Paty's first time. He had done so for several years. He was always careful as it was against France's law to identify anyone by their religion. He warned his pupils at the start that they could look away if they thought they might be offended. The first caricature showed the Prophet Muhammad holding a 'Je Suis Charlie' sign. It was deemed blasphemous to Muslims for giving him a face. The second caricature was Muhammad on all fours, naked, with a star emerging from his backside and the caption 'A star is born!'.

Once his pupils had seen the drawings he would explain how French law protected them, as part of freedom of speech enshrined in the Republic.

According to reports, one filed a complaint to the police. He also posted a video on Facebook to mobilise others, identifying who the teacher was and calling him a thug. 'He should no longer teach our children. He should go and educate himself.' A known Islamist agitator, Abdelhakim Sefrioui, came to the school and made a video decrying 'irresponsible and aggressive behaviour'. The school and police authorities supported Paty, saying he had followed correct classroom procedure. No disciplinary action. Paty took action and a defamation complaint against the parent who had abused him. The law, he thought, was on his side.

The French president, Emmanuel Macron responded by saying the beheading was an attack on 'the republic and its values'. Four people, including a minor, are reported to have been arrested since.

In France, the education system includes obligatory courses, one of them being 'moral and civil education' where free speech is fundamental. According to reports by *The Guardian*, 'After the contested lesson, an angry parent posted a video on YouTube complaining about the teacher.' On Friday night, another parent posted below the video, defending the professor, writing: 'I am a parent of a student at this college. The teacher just showed caricatures from *Charlie Hebdo* as part of a history lesson on freedom of expression. He asked the Muslim students to leave the classroom if they wished, out of respect . . . He was a great teacher. He tried to encourage the critical spirit of his students, always with respect and intelligence. This evening, I am sad, for my daughter, but also for teachers in France. Can we continue to teach without being afraid of being killed?"

The video was taken down on Friday night. Abdoullakh Anzorov, eighteen, a Chechen national living in France since the age of six, was arrested. Anzorov was already riled after the teacher showed one of his high school classes a series of caricatures, including one of the Prophet Muhammad, during a lesson on free speech.

After his death, French police raided dozens of suspected Islamist groups and individuals accused of extremism. Among them, high-profile Muslim organisations including the Collective for the Fight Against Islamophobia in France (CCIF) and Barakacity a humanitarian organisation that has carried out projects in Togo, southeast Asia and Pakistan.

The French interior minister, Gérard Darmanin, said the CCIF was implicated in the murder of Paty as a video posted on Facebook implicated it in what he described as a 'fatwa' against the history teacher.

'It is an Islamist outfit that does not condemn the attacks . . . that has invited radical islamists. It is an agency against the republic. It considers there is a state of Islamophobia all the while being subsidized (financially) by the French state. And I think it's time we stopped being naive with these outfits on our territory,' he told *Libération*.

Darmanin has overseen raids on Islamic organisations and individuals, and went as far as to criticise supermarkets over their separate halal and kosher sections, defending the police actions, insisting France was seeking to stamp out extremism.

Fire fire burning bright, in the forests of the night

'We are seeking to fight an ideology, not a religion. I think the great majority of French Muslims are well aware they are the first affected by the ideological drift of radical Islam,' Darmanin told *Libération*.

Macron, defending the nation's liberty of free speech declared that France would not 'renounce the caricatures'. Iranian officials based in France felt the response was 'unwise'. A report on state TV claimed an official from the Iranian foreign ministry in Tehran had accused France of fostering hatred against Islam under the guise of freedom of expression.

Reports from various sources compiled by *The Guardian* are as follows:

> A powerful association of clerics in the Iranian city of Qom, also urged the country's government to condemn Macron's remarks and called on Islamic nations to impose political and economic sanctions on France. One hardline Iranian newspaper depicted the French president as the devil, portraying him as Satan in a cartoon on its front page.
>
> In Saudi Arabia, the country's state run press agency quoted an anonymous foreign ministry official saying the kingdom 'rejects any attempt to link Islam and terrorism, and denounces the offensive cartoons of the prophet'.
>
> In Bangladesh, an estimated 40,000 people took part in an anti-France rally in the capital, Dhaka, burning an effigy of Macron and calling for a boycott of French products. The rally was organized by Islami Andolan Bangladesh (IAB), one of the

country's largest Islamist parties. There were also calls for the Bangladeshi government to order the French ambassador back to Paris and threats to tear down the French embassy building.

Within a month since Paty's murder, three assault cases occurred in France. All linked to free speech. 'If we are under attack, it's for our values, for our taste for liberty.' Macron said to the nation in Nice, 'I want to say to all citizens, whether they practice a religion or not, that we are one.'

The fourth and seventh prime minister of Malaysia Tun Dr Mahathir Mohamad had this to say on his blog and twitter accounts just hours after the third assault in Paris:

1. A teacher in France had his throat slit by an 18-year-old Chechen boy. The killer was angered by the teacher showing a caricature of Prophet Muhammad. The teacher intended to demonstrate freedom of expression.

2. The killing is not an act that as a Muslim I would approve. But while I believe in the freedom of expression, I do not think it includes insulting other people. You cannot go up to a man and curse him simply because you believe in freedom of speech.

3. In Malaysia, where there are people of many different races and religions, we have avoided serious conflicts between races because we are conscious of the need to be sensitive to the sensitivities of others. If we are not, then this country would never be peaceful and stable.

4. We often copy the ways of the West. We dress like them, we adopt their political systems, even some of their strange practices. But we have our own values, different as between races and religions, which we need to sustain.

5. The trouble with new ideas is that the late comers tend to add new interpretations. These are not what the originators intended. Thus, freedom for women meant the right to vote in elections. Today, we want to eliminate everything that is different between men and women.

6. Physically we are different. This limits our capacity to be equal. We have to accept these differences and the limitations that are placed on us. Our value system is also a part of human rights.

7. Yes, sometimes some values seem to be inhuman. They cause some people to suffer. We need to reduce the suffering.
   But not by force, if the resistance is great.

8. The dress code of European women at one time was severely restrictive. Apart from the face no part of the body was exposed. But over the years, more and more parts of the body are exposed. Today a little string covers the most secret place, that's all. In fact, many in the west are totally naked when on certain beaches.

9. The West accepts this as normal. But the West should not try to forcibly impose this on others. To do so is to deprive the freedom of these people.

10. Generally, the west no longer adhere to their own religion. They are Christians in name only. That is their right. But they must not show disrespect for the values of others, for the religion of others. It is a measure of the level of their civilization to show this respect.

11. Macron is not showing that he is civilised. He is very primitive in blaming the religion of Islam and Muslims for the killing of the insulting school teacher. It is not in keeping with the teachings of Islam. But irrespective of the religion professed, angry people kill. The French in the course of their history have killed millions of people. Many were Muslims.

12. Muslims have a right to be angry and to kill millions of French people for the massacres of the past. But by and large the Muslims have not applied the 'eye for an eye' law. Muslims don't. The French shouldn't. Instead the French should teach their people to respect other people's feelings.

13. Since you have blamed all Muslims and the Muslims' religion for what was done by one angry person, the Muslims have a right to punish the French. The boycott cannot compensate for the wrongs committed by the French all these years.

Twitter flagged it for instigating violence.

A Pound of flesh for a pound of flesh, an aye for an aye

As one of Europe's colonial powerhouse, France has never been without its tapestry of violence. *Charlie Hebdo's* satirical magazine and their extol for free speech is no different to Homer's *Cyclops* and one optic.

In Homer's words:

> An overweening and lawless folk, who, trusting in the immortal gods, plant nothing with their hands nor plough; but all these things spring up for them without sowing or ploughing, wheat, and barley, and vines, which bear the rich clusters of wine, and the rain of Zeus gives them increase. Neither assemblies for council have they, nor appointed laws, but they dwell on the peaks of lofty mountains in hollow caves, and each one is lawgiver to his children and his wives, and they wreck nothing one of another.

This is not to say the French are uncivilized. But in their unwavering pursuit for free speech, they could be suffering from myopia. There is a reason why the cyclopes have one eye which makes them consequently uncivilized shepherds. They represent people who see through only one perspective. And this won't be a coincidence for the French. Perhaps it is psychological conditioning.

'In the colonial context the settler only ends his work of breaking in the native when the latter admits loudly and intelligibly the supremacy of the white man's values.'

Frantz Fanon, *The Wretched of the Earth*

In 1961, Fanon published a book called *Les Damnés de la Terre* (*The Wretched of the Earth*). *The Wretched of the Earth* is Fanon's psychiatric

51

and psychological analysis of the dehumanizing effects of colonization upon the individual and the nation. Published just before Fanon's death, *The Wretched of the Earth* is a seminal read written with the Algerian independence struggle in mind. Prefaced by Jean Paul Sartre, the book offers a social-psychological analysis of colonialism, continuing his argument that there is a deep connection between colonialism and the mind, and equally between colonial war and mental disease.

Fanon was black. Everyday he endured racism. It was a relentless war, a persistent disease. There was no way out of it, he noted. In *The Wretched,* Fanon argued for violent revolution against colonial control, ending in socialism. These struggles must be combined, he argued with (re)building national culture, and in that sense Fanon was a supporter of socialist nationalism. In the book, Fanon not only writes about violence in the international context, colonialism, national consciousness and freedom fighting, but he also includes a psychoanalytic investigation of mental disorders associated with colonial war. The book, then, continues his work of drawing connections between the inner world of subjugated individuals and the workings of international politics. This is something that has been continued by other scholars in the postcolonial tradition including Ashis Nandy and Ngũgĩ wa Thiong'o.

To Fanon, colonialism will never permanently exit the realm of command and conquer. And to countries and people who have been colonized by a European supremacy, while physical oppression may go away and be replaced by independence, mental imperialism persists. The bully will forever position to dominate and the oppressed will either take into another form of oppressor or debase itself to a lower level of subjugation.

> How come he cannot recognize his own cruelty now turned against him? How come he can't see his own savagery as a colonist in the savagery of these oppressed peasants who have absorbed it through every pore and for which they can find no cure? The answer is simple: this arrogant individual, whose power of authority and fear of losing it has gone to his head, has difficulty remembering he was once a man; he thinks he is a whip or a gun; he is convinced that the domestication

of the 'inferior races' is obtained by governing their reflexes. He disregards the human memory, the indelible reminders; and then, above all, there is this that perhaps he never know: we only become what we are by radically negating deep down what others have done to us.

Jean-Paul Sartre, *The Wretched of the Earth*

Thinkers around the globe have been profoundly influenced by Fanon's work on anti-black racism and decolonization theory. Brazilian theorist of critical pedagogy Paulo Freire engages Fanon in dialogue in *Pedagogy of the Oppressed*, notably in his discussion of the missteps that oppressed people may make on their path to liberation. Freire's emphasis on the need to go beyond a mere turning of the tables, a seizure of the privileges and social positions of the oppressors, echoes Fanon's concern in *Les Damnés* and in essays such as 'Racism and Culture' (in *Pour la Révolution Africaine*), that failure to appreciate the deeply Manichean structure of the settler-native division could lead to a false decolonization in which a native elite simply replace the settler elite as the oppressive rulers of the still-exploited masses. This shared concern is the motivation for Freire's insistence on perspectival transformation and on populist inclusion as necessary conditions for social liberation.

Race, race. It was always about race.
The kind no one wins

'We didn't start the fire
It was always burning
Since the world's been turning'
Billy Joel, *We didn't start the fire* (1989)

As a student of journalism, history is like *The Da Vinci Code*. History speaks volume about the future while shrouding a past that could shatter humanity. History contains pieces of puzzles to help you unlock many bigger mysteries. Symbols aplenty raising speculations, the building blocks for conspiracy theorists. COVID-19 is touted as one. A cabal orchestrates world domination to profit huge pharmas, melt the permafrost of a global economy to incite a new open market for nascent industries and products. A paradigm shift. This is not the strength of everyone's daily cup of tea so the powers that be decide to water it down and call it 'the new normal'.

Meanwhile, the killing of Samuel Paty has triggered religious disputes the world over. Below is an article difficult to refute.

Reprinting the *Charlie Hebdo* cartoons is not about free speech

It is about using speech to reaffirm domination.

By Asma Barlas posted on *Al Jazeera* on 10 September 2020.

French satirical magazine *Charlie Hebdo* is at it, again: it has chosen to republish the derogatory cartoons of Prophet Muhammad which provoked a violent attack against it in 2015. The editors say it is 'essential' to reprint these on the eve of the trial of the perpetrators of that violence.

A decade earlier, in 2005, the Danish newspaper *Morgenavisen Jyllands-Posten* also published a dozen defamatory cartoons of the prophet which it then republished three years later.

It was the printing of these cartoons that ultimately provoked some Muslims to resort to violence and, as is customary, it was their backlash that became the nub of the 'cartoon controversy'.

The original affront to Muslim religious sensibilities was swallowed up by assertions of the cartoonists' right to free speech and to engage in humour. In fact, in most critics' views, it was not just the cartoonists who were victimised by 'Islamic rage,' but also the principle of free speech itself.

However, it should be possible to condemn violence by Muslims without giving a free pass to those who defame and vilify their religion, their prophet and their scripture. Yet, this rarely happens.

Instead, the Muslim-baiting intelligentsia relies on precisely its own vilifications to incite the violence which it then feigns to be horrified and surprised by. I say feigns because, by now, pretty much everyone knows that, goaded to a point, some Muslims will respond violently to caricatures of their prophet as a terrorist, among other things. I also say feigns because provocateurs require such a response to anathematise all Muslims as a threat to European identities and values.

If it is easy enough to understand why some Muslims respond violently to derogatory tropes about Islam, the prophet and the Quran, what does it say about those who compulsively keep recycling these? I have speculated about this need at length elsewhere but will make only some brief points here.

First, it is difficult to see how anyone—not only a Muslim— could find a cartoon of the prophet as a terrorist/suicide bomber amusing without also treating terrorism itself lightly. After all, how many of us can laugh at a cartoon of a suicide bomber, irrespective of who that person is supposed to be? As for the purported irony of such representations of the prophet, what is satirical about these, when Muslims are already viewed as born terrorists-in-the-making?

Second, European vilifications of the prophet and Islam have a much older pedigree than free speech and have nothing to do with humour. To be precise, they have their roots in medieval Europe and the changing self-conceptions of Christians over a millennium.

For instance, Tomaz Mastnak, a historian of the Crusades, argues that it was in the mid-ninth century when Western unity began to express itself as Christendom, that Muslims also came to be seen as the 'normative enemies' of Christianity. Until then, they had been viewed as just another pagan group and generally ignored—even the Muslim conquest of southern Spain did not make it into leading chronicles.

Over time though, Europe's Christians came to see in Islam not just a 'sinister conspiracy against Christianity [but] that total negation of [it] ... which would mark the contrivances of Antichrist'. This is how Robert Southern describes it in his book *Western Views of Islam* in the Middle Ages and he attributes this suspicion to the 'strong desire not to know [Islam] for fear of contamination'.

Instead, he says, even the Christians who lived in 'the middle of Islam' (Muslim-ruled Andalusia) looked to the Bible to explain it, which is how they came to consider it the Antichrist. In short, according to Southern, it was ignorance and the fear of contamination that made 'the existence of Islam the most far-reaching problem in medieval Christendom'.

Given this history, it is not surprising that medieval Christians would also portray the prophet as a heathen idol, the devil, Mahound (as in Salman Rushdie's *Satanic Verses*), an imposter, and the Antichrist. He appears in such guises from the Crusades to the Reformation, with his representation as a religious imposter, reaching its literary apotheosis in Italian poet Dante Alighieri's *Divine Comedy*, in which he is confined to the eighth circle of hell.

Two centuries later, he reappears as an Antichrist in the work of German reformist Martin Luther, who of course, believed the pope and the Catholic Church were much worse. A century later, Dutch jurist Hugo Grotius, lauded as the father of international law, was still calling him 'a robber' and declaring that, in contrast to the Christians, who 'were men who feared God, and led innocent lives… they who first embraced Mahometanism were robbers, and men void of humanity and piety'.

With the coming of the Enlightenment, the prophet's critics also began assailing him in secular language, as the 'worst type of … fanatic' (French writer Voltaire) and 'the greatest enemy of reason who ever lived' (German philosopher Immanuel Kant).

Such depictions did not, however, portend a change in his representation as the antithesis of European civilisation. If he was no longer called an Antichrist, in European minds, he was still thought to be outside reason and rationality. This is why I see the cartoons of the prophet as a terrorist to be just a secularisation of the figure of the Antichrist.

Both images serve, equally powerfully, to locate him and, by extension, Islam and Muslims as Europe's natural enemies. This is why reducing the cartoons to just an issue of free speech obscures their historical and ideological genealogy.

Lastly, (free) speech is conducive not only to critique, humour, honesty, and dissent but also to assertions of dominance and enactments of power. Though power is enacted differently, its exercise is 'inseparable from its display', as American writer Saidiya Hartman argues in her book *Terror, Slavery, and Self-Making in Nineteenth-Century America.*

In the context of slavery in North America, for instance, being able to represent power was 'essential to reproducing domination'. As an example, Hartman notes that a slave-holder's 'display of mastery [over a slave] was just as important as the legal title to slave property'. This display usually involved demonstrating the slave holder's 'dominion and the captive's abasement,' publicly. It also took the less obtrusive form of organising 'innocent amusements and spectacles of mastery' as a way for the dominant classes 'to establish their dominion' over the enslaved and dominated.

Borrowing from Hartman, I want to suggest that, today, some Westerners seek to demonstrate and reproduce their dominion over Muslims by caricaturing and maligning our sacred symbols at will. They are thus able to achieve epistemically what they cannot physically or legally. Even if this displacement from the physical to the psychological signifies the limits of Western power, speech is integral to its display. This is why derogatory caricatures of the prophet function as spectacles of mastery and as an ideological means to bolster intra-Western unity against Muslims.

It is as much to such enactments of mastery as it is to the content of specific attacks that Muslims like myself react angrily, and what we condemn is not the idea that people should be free to speak but the use of speech to dominate and degrade the already marginal or vulnerable. Defending domination in the name of freedom just confirms that not all conceptions of freedom are equally worth defending.

The views expressed in this article are the author's own and do not necessarily reflect Al Jazeera's editorial stance.

The otherness of facts and fiction

Barlas' piece was not the first and won't be the last to touch on the abuse of freedom, and how historical context is key to the discourse. More importantly, how impartial are we to the annals of history? Dan Brown through his investigative series from *Angels and Demons, The Da Vinci Code* to *The Lost Symbol*, often made allusions that the Vatican held ancient secrets that conspired to select parts of Christianity that served its patriarchal purpose. This includes the battle of the Crusades where it was the Christians that were robbed of significant knowledge and science. And thus, the binary opposition of good and bad between the Christians and the Muslims have been ingrained ever since. So it has come to be known that every state must have its enemy, every dispute an opponent, and every religion its anti-Christ.

Edward Said describes this problem as 'Orientalism'. Orientalism is a way of seeing, that imagines, emphasizes, exaggerates and distorts differences of Arab peoples and cultures as compared to that of Europe and the West. It often involves seeing Arab culture as exotic, backward, uncivilized, and at times dangerous. Coupled with colonialism's arrogance and power for domination, prejudiced outsider interpretation will continue to be a stumbling block for future democracy. As Said states with eloquence in *Culture and Imperialism*:

> No one today is purely one thing. Labels like Indian, or woman, or Muslim, or American are not more than starting-points, which if followed into actual experience for only a moment are quickly left behind. Imperialism consolidated the mixture of cultures and identities on a global scale. But its worst and most paradoxical

gift was to allow people to believe that they were only, mainly, exclusively, white, or Black, or Western, or Oriental. Yet just as human beings make their own history, they also make their cultures and ethnic identities. No one can deny the persisting continuities of long traditions, sustained habitations, national languages, and cultural geographies, but there seems no reason except fear and prejudice to keep insisting on their separation and distinctiveness, as if that was all human life was about. Survival in fact is about the connections between things; in Eliot's phrase, reality cannot be deprived of the 'other echoes [that] inhabit the garden.' It is more rewarding—and more difficult—to think concretely and sympathetically, contrapuntally, about others than only about 'us.' But this also means not trying to rule others, not trying to classify them or put them in hierarchies, above all, not constantly reiterating how 'our' culture or country is number one (or not number one, for that matter).

Free speech itself is an abused concept, if not a figurative speech. And modern governments have wrestled its arm, a constitutional victim of prejudiced outsider-and-insider interpretation.

Even Shakespeare teased the idea of a pound of flesh for a pound of flesh. Never intended for literal translation, it was an intention of value spoken by Shylock, a shrewd Jew with a contempt for Christians. Shakespeare coined the figure of speech to refer to a lawful but unreasonable recompense during the sixteenth century. The flesh suggests vengeful, bloodthirstiness, and inflexible behaviour to get back borrowed money. This was followed by the concept of mercy linked with the Christian idea of salvation.

This phrase is a figurative method of expressing a spiteful penalty or a harsh demand, the consequences of non-payment on a distressed bargain. However, the usurer Shylock asks for a real pound of flesh as security when merchant Antonio comes and borrows money. Antonio accepts the brutal terms of Shylock, but he is aware of the fact that Shylock despises him. In a twist of misfortune, Antonio cannot pay back Shylock's money. Coincidentally, Shylock too has had a twist of misfortune. Now filled with desperation and increasing contempt, demands his flesh as a fine.

Ultimately, Antonio is forced to default, while the usurer refuses the merchant's beg for mercy. Dressed as a famous judge, and an indirect beneficiary of Antonio, Portia takes a letter of bond on the insistence of Shylock and brings an absurd conclusion. She maintains that the bond specifies a pound of flesh but 'no jot of blood'. Using wit and legal sophistry Portia, offers a solution: Should a single drop of Christian blood be shed after cutting his flesh, then under Venetian law, the state of Venice would take away Shylock's property and land. Antonio is spared and the story ends with a celebration.

Perhaps the idea of free speech has always been false advertising. A deception. After all, while freedom of speech is a fundamental right, it is not absolute. Everything and anything we say, can and will be used against us because context is subject to restriction, dissection and interpretation. Today, it's also about intergeneration.

As a Malaysian I read and reread my former premier's public condemnation. I see an intergenerational concern rooted in education. Tun Dr Mahathir Mohamad speaks from a different generation. A generation that studied the Algerian massacres and the French colonisation (note: these topics are not covered in today's secular education in Malaysia). Recorded history shows the French were brutal to the Muslims as the Dutch were to the Indonesians and South Africa. Second problem is that we teach history and the constitution at a very superficial level in schools (superficial that it leaves no cognitive impression) that at the rate of things, everything becomes an emotional attack, a succession of putting out fires and categorised under extremism.

All killings are unacceptable regardless of intent. That is the rule of law. All life is of equal value. A pound of flesh to a pound of flesh. It is a travesty of law when a life is executed without rightful trial and when dissenting citizens are made to disappear. Liberté, égalité, fraternité.

The French themselves have had a tumultuous history soldiering through the French revolution, surviving the razor edge of the guillotine hence why they extol their freedom of speech more than Malaysians can understand. As the Sapir-Whorf hypothesis would suggest: we can't prescribe what hasn't been ascribed.

But we can disagree, just don't disrespect. It boils down to ethics.

In political theory, Aristotle is famous for observing that 'man is a political animal,' meaning that human beings naturally form political communities. Human beings cannot thrive outside a community or exist as an island. The basic purpose of communities is to promote human flourishing. Aristotle devised a classification of forms of government.

According to Aristotle, states may be classified according to the number of their rulers and the interests in which they govern. Rule by one person in the interest of all is monarchy; rule by one person in his own interest is tyranny. Rule by a minority in the interest of all is aristocracy; rule by a minority in the interest of itself is oligarchy. Rule by a majority in the interest of all is 'polity'; rule by a majority in its own interest is 'democracy.' In theory, the best form of government is monarchy, and the next best is aristocracy. However, because monarchy and aristocracy frequently devolve into tyranny and oligarchy, respectively, in practice the best form is polity.

His definition of democracy was unpopular, considered unusual and was never widely accepted.

Religion and politics have always been deemed taboo in all social discourses as they are open to interpretation. To expect solidarity of thought would be naiveté. But ground rules aren't impossible. All leaders as a rule should practice ethics of diplomacy where words that you say should uplift and unite, to promote the pursuit of happiness, not incite for division. As much as history has brought us to where we are, the aim is to be change-makers. And while we may not be able to bleach our past we can attempt to break generational curses. As Søren Kierkegaard wrote: 'Life can only be understood backwards; but it must be lived forwards'.

The one marvel I have for COVID-19 is despite the havoc it has created, it unites us to pay attention to a universal truth: we need to rebuild ourselves. Perhaps it is time to unlearn and relearn.

Liberté, Egalité, Fraternité.

A World on fire: Of fraying politics and broken economies

'Hearts are worn in these dark ages
You're not alone in this story's pages
The light has fallen amongst the living and the dying
And I'll try to hold it in, yeah, I'll try to hold it in

The world's on fire, it's more than I can handle
Tap into the water, try to bring my share
Try to bring more, more than I can handle
Bring it to the table, bring what I am able

I watch the heavens but I find no calling
Something I can do to change what's coming
Stay close to me while the sky is falling
I don't wanna be left alone, don't wanna be alone

The world's on fire, it's more than I can handle'
Sarah McLachlan, *World on Fire* from the album *Afterglow* (2003)

In October 2020, we experienced a second wave of the coronavirus. A spike would often signify another lockdown.

This round, shopping malls were the red zones. We all knew a second wave was imminent but after months of prior lockdown we had expected the government to have a contingency plan to mitigate the spread. We were wrong on that account.

It was then announced that 14-27 October will be a second conditional movement control order (CMCO).

Hopes were crushed. Once again, the wings of our freedom were to be clipped.

The lockdown operating procedures were reinstated: Schools closed; only two per household allowed to go out; Grab can only take maximum two passengers per ride; many diners closed for in-house seating; no interstate travelling except for work and emergencies with official documents. And then it got worse.

On November 7, Senior Minister Datuk Seri Ismail Sabri Yaakob said all states in Peninsular Malaysia, except for Perlis, Pahang and Kelantan, will be placed under the conditional movement control order for four weeks from November 9 to December 6. For the Klang Valley populace, this was an additional length and people were already hanging by the skin of their teeth. Many were disappointed especially after we had begun to savour a taste of normalcy after the first CMCO was uplifted in August. At the rate of things, it looks like we will be toasting the new year in our living rooms.

But why was this second lockdown a bigger bummer for us all? Shouldn't we be more concerned about the resurgence of the coronavirus? Shouldn't we be more equipped at handling these situations compared to the first? This isn't a shocker, but why did it rob our motivation even worse? Goleman writes, 'Life is a comedy for those who think and a tragedy for those who feel.' Perhaps it is best to feel less. But it is inescapable when often it felt like we were dancing on fire.

Foray, Stray and into the Grey

'Cognitive dissonance is the motivational mechanism that underlies the reluctance to admit mistakes or accept scientific findings even when those findings can save our lives.'
Leon Festinger, social psychologist

There were days I was engrossed with world affairs, fascinated with what was happening, but there were also days I totally lost it and wanted to capture a wandering thought or a memory that popped up.

Cognitive dissonance. I admit, in the first eight months I thought COVID was a hoax. Reading into Agenda 21[1] about a speculated 'depopulation project' I thought I was part of a huge conspiracy orchestrated by a cabal led by the world's most powerful and distinguished.

Then in February 2021 my partner collapsed in his home in Bangkok. Few days earlier, he had complained of breathing problems. Chest heavy with shortness of breath, we suspected pneumonia linked to his asthma. On two separate occasions, he had taken the COVID swab tests and results came back negative. This time, however, he was isolated immediately and placed in the intensive care unit confirmed for COVID-19. Contact tracing showed he was infected from a passenger while on a business flight from Chiang Mai to Bangkok. The passenger reportedly died after a few days while my partner was in ICU for three weeks, and remains in respiratory rehabilitation up to this day due to scarring of the lungs. Being separated and swimming in anxiety for

---

[1] Agenda 21 was raised in 1992 at the first International Earth Summit at Rio de Janeiro, Brazil. It aimed to combat environmental damage, poverty disease through global cooperation.

weeks felt like eternity. The five weeks he was in hospital dependent on ventilators made me reflect on what I really thought and felt about COVID-19 minus all the media reports, hearsay and speculation. It wasn't always easy.

It was during these punishing moments that I often slipped in and out of global affairs and into random thoughts. Many etched memories I felt were perhaps my way of emotional justice, a way to hold multiple truths at a time where we had to recognize, validate and respond to many realities. A part of me remains skeptical of COVID-19, another accepts, a portion indulges in the mounting conspiracies on why this is happening. I suppose we are as thirsty for the truth as we are to be entertained.

While journalling to support my sanity, I often reeled back to my university days. Days that compared to today were simpler because writing was one undertaking my English Literature professors made compulsory. Much to their chagrin, I often wrote about Sigmund Freud, father of psychoanalysis. Controversial, sexist, and as W. H. Auden once commented, 'a climate of opinion.' Now that I'm in COVID purgatory, I am thankful for those requisitions. Penning these fleeting thoughts is cathartic, offers respite and relief I couldn't get from talking with another COVID sufferer without drowning in their own subjugation of pity and fear.

> Much like COVID-19 and its strains of mutation, Freud was always a step ahead of the prudish Victorian thinkers. In surreal fashion, it was also Freud who said, 'One day, in retrospect, the years of struggle will strike you as the most beautiful.' How apt this is in our current time of corona. Back in the late nineties as a rebelling adolescent delving into philosophy, nothing was more striking than this Freudian point of view. 'I have found little that is good in human beings on the whole. In my experience most of them are trash, no matter whether they publicly subscribe to this or that ethical doctrine or to none at all. That is something you cannot say aloud, or perhaps even think.'

Freud was the James Dean of nineteenth century intellectual discourse. In the early 1900s when Freud published *Interpretation of Dreams*, he received criticism for describing problems of the human psyche based on conversations he had had with patients. 'The dream is the liberation of the spirit from the pressure of external nature, a detachment of the soul from the fetters of matter.' Not exactly hard science. Where is the research to back his theories, his combatants asked.

Freud stood by his work vehemently and had loyal supporters. To prove his prowess, psychology remains the only scientific field in modern medicine that deals with its patients via conversations, including prescribing medication prior to physical testing. His followers, most notably Carl Jung, helped to expand notions of his work into cross disciplines. Perhaps in due time, like COVID-19, we will incrementally understand what Freud saw that others couldn't:

> Humanity has in the course of time had to endure from the hands of science two great outrages upon its naive self-love. The first was when we realized that our earth was not the center of the universe, but only a tiny speck in a world-system of a magnitude hardly conceivable; this is associated in our minds with the name of Copernicus, although Alexandrian doctrines taught something very similar. The second was when biological research robbed man of his peculiar privilege of having been specially created, and relegated him to a descent from the animal world, implying an ineradicable animal nature in him: this transvaluation has been accomplished in our own time upon the instigation of Charles Darwin, Wallace, and their predecessors, and not without the most violent opposition from their contemporaries. But man's craving for grandiosity is now suffering the third and most bitter blow from present-day psychological research which is endeavoring to prove to the ego of each one of us that he is not even master in his own house, but that he must remain content with the veriest scraps of information about what is going on unconsciously in his own mind. We psycho-analysts were neither the first nor the only ones to propose to mankind that they should look inward; but it appears to be our lot to advocate it most insistently and to support it by empirical evidence which touches every man closely.
> Sigmund Freud, *Introduction à la psychanalyse*

I used to feel intimidated when people asked about my qualifications. When it comes to my work discussing creative art and human behaviour, I had neither a PhD nor a litany of published work in high impact journals. I have, however, 16 years of first hand experiences teaching and learning creativity and communications rooted in the Waldorf method. What would Freud say? Today, looking at the media and the COVID brouhaha I remind myself, if Bill Gates has no formal education in medicine yet is part of a global vaccination mandate, I'm just as qualified as he is. What is important, according to Freud, is a curious and wandering mind. Be like a poet, Freud opined. 'Poets are masters of us ordinary men, in knowledge of the mind, because they drink at streams which we have not yet made accessible to science.' Curious, wandering and poetic, that I was. I recall a moment in time.

I was 21 at university when my creative writing lecturer suggested I publish.

Why? I asked.

'Because you should write for others,' he replied.

'But I write for myself.'

'Then you should reconsider. Some writers, when they write, they can inspire. All writings should. And you should be one of them.'

'Should.' That is an interesting choice of words, I thought. 'It's not really what I had in mind to do with myself.'

'Well, what are your plans?'

'Well sir, I'm thinking of studying behavioural sciences and applying to Quantico. Criminal profiling and crime scene investigation are what I have in mind. I'd like to join the Federal Bureau of Investigation.'

'Well then, even more so you should seriously consider becoming a writer. Writing alone won't be enough. You should publish!'

'But sir, I was thinking . . . '

'Right there, is your talent. You're creative and with a sense of humour. The world needs more tongue-in-cheek writers.'

'I was serious about the FBI thing sir . . . '

'Your first article should be The 10 Commandments on How to be a Good Writer.'

'Why that sir? Doesn't sound very exciting. A bit too elementary, no?'

'Consider it a self-boosting exercise. By writing out the ten steps you're teaching others and reminding yourself what it takes to be a good writer.'

'Perhaps a tweak in the idea sir?'

'Like what?'

'Ten Ways To Identify A Serial Killer.'

There was an awkward silence between my professor and I. He blinked a few times. Adolescents do not react well in silence. 'Father Freud said, neurosis is the inability to tolerate ambiguity.'

Mysticism and Madness

Reading the coronavirus chronicles in the *New Yorker,* the mask mandate remains a fascinating topic of human stubbornness and of tribal defiance. In fact, all over the world, the response to the public health crisis reveals a stark divide over how to get life back to normal. The truth is, seeking normal is arguably the problem.

Writes Atul Gawande, 'Everyday seems to bring another test of whether our democracy can succeed in managing the problems of a country . . . big, varied and individualistic . . . ' And that's true. The more developed we become, the more contentious. We elect leaders to represent us only to doubt, question and persecute them. Granted they are usually corrupted but within systems we create, and once sucked into the knots of power, difficult to untangle. Perhaps, it's because we put too much faith in people, and the coronavirus is a reminder that what we do not see is what will define us. This helps to explain why despite the experts in the world and repeated viral outbreaks throughout history, we are still without a cohesive strategic plan that prepares us for a pandemic.

Ironically this circuitry of deviating behaviour has been an ancient practice with a high fatality rate.

Since the dawn of man's existence, humans have lived in a tribal community setting anchored to the concept of totemism.

Totemism is a system of belief in which humans are said to have kinship or a mystical relationship with a spirit-being, such as an animal or plant. The entity, or totem, is thought to interact with a given kin group or an individual and to serve as their emblem or symbol.

In 1927, Freud brought to light totemism stating it was a crucial concept that held communities together like glue. In fact on several occasions throughout his life's work, Freud affirmed that psychoanalysis, acts like totemism, is a 'bridge,' a 'link in a chain,' or rather, that it promises to be one, and in so doing acquires a mediating function between the medical sciences, psychopathology and the sciences of the mind, and the sciences of culture.

The goal in life via totemism? To strive for meaning, hopefulness and purpose.

A village is said to encompass every component of life; farmer, blacksmith, fisherman, midwife, musicians, artisans, shaman. A blending of the real and the esoteric. This becomes an ecosystem of wellness. What you need, someone has the skills to provide. Everyone is a neighbour away and life is a shared experience. In Borneo, the Rumah Panjang is a perfect example. And it becomes a witness to all as each member grows, evolves and in spiritual terms, we call this transformative.

Everyone functions accordingly, until someone sticks out. The '*Gong*', says the people of Terengganu, refers to the creative, or the madman. In reflection of Freud's totemism ideology, this becomes problematic as 'the individual (or individualism) is essentially an enemy of society and has instinctual urges that must be restrained to help society function. Among these instinctual wishes are those of incest, cannibalism, and lust for killing.' Extreme, perhaps, but today these are the tropes and staples of modern horror entertainment fare.

Identically when a person experiences a psychological distress and alienation, which are normal occurrences, he is said to be disconnected from oneself and the community. In today's terms, we call this mental illness. And while the word mental is positive, the word illness is perceived as negative.

The tradition is that a journey for meaning and purpose is a spiritual journey (made even more famous by Paulo Coelho and the concept of Hero's Journey). A spiritual journey is a transformative experience. Being ritualistic makes it mystical because every transformative experience carries with it, its own history and language. It is through the presence of orthodox religion that such experiences are described as self-delusion, uncritical superstition, raising issues of authority.

Similar to this is the chronicles of the Salem witch-hunts. If you had a mole, a birthmark, a social dissonance of some sort, you were burnt at the stake for witchcraft. This was made worse with the intervention of religion and its divisiveness towards what the Church disagreed with, meaning all forms of unrepresentativeness was demonic by nature.

Today this has become a clusterfuck.

One can't tell if a wayward leader, attempting to placate COVID chaos, is a *Gong*, a maverick, or an impending disaster. Is he being eccentric, a creative anomaly, or a totem?

Perhaps this is all Freud's fault. And for a former disciple of Freudism, this is not an easy confession.

Freud was the *Gong* of the nineteenth century. What helped to exacerbate his theories was the zeitgeist of the industrial revolution. As infrastructure for modern transportation progressed, so was people's curiosity for the world. His *Interpretation of Dreams* (1899) picked on an existing scab of our human consciousness, sub and unconsciousness. But it was his book *The Future of an Illusion* (1927) that took a Marxist sword and sliced through the fat of Catholicism. Riding on Karl Marx's 'religion being the opiate of the masses' shibboleth, Freud tore down the house of worship by describing religious impulses as mystical impulses, being not only the universal compulsive neurosis of mankind, but rooted in narcissistic needs, attachments and wish fulfilments. The medical fraternity grew ambivalent towards the mystical impulse of the human person ever since. Today I can't tell this from a politician, much alone to trust one handling the vaccine negotiation and distribution. After all, this whole COVID debacle is as mystical as it comes.

Accused of lacking in judicious evidence, mystical experience is so ambiguous that it is difficult to be measured by what comforts modern thinkers rooted in empirical evidence: structured questionnaires.

And here we return to Freud. Like his theories for *Interpretation of Dreams*, self-reports were the only reliable source of evidence on what is happening in a transformative experience. Self-reports of ecstatic divine union was one indicator that the person is having a mystical experience.

After such an episode, the person is never the same.

As all transformative experiences go, perceptual changes occur. In some cases, the perceptual change in experience leads to increasing fragmentation and confusion. Hence, a popular term is coined: *psychosis*. And from there, modern madness was born.

I am writing this as being in lockdown has indeed been a transformative experience. Sometimes I feel it spirals into psychosis. The virus is a totem that has glued the world without revealing itself only its devastating effects and mutating prowess. All I can do to protect myself is to wear a mask and pray for luck.

As much as I would like to persecute the leaders and burn them at the stake for their lack of governing skills, I must also stop and remind myself that perhaps, and this has to be underlined, highlighted, and uppercased, they're a *Gong* with abilities I cannot comprehend. In my ignorance, I am therefore made irate and frustrated.

Perhaps mayhem is magic.

Perhaps, if we allow ourselves to be roasted in the mysteries of this virus we can learn to enjoy this pandemic as we see whatever that unfolds as transformative. Have we all spiraled into psychosis?

There is only so much that we can control. If people could come together to support a mystical relationship with a spirit-being, fondly known as religion, why can't we overcome a virus?

Has the media become an instigator for our COVID psychosis? Has religion?

The US Presidential Election and Batman

It is November 2020.

Months leading up to November, media posts and airplay dedicated most of its reporting on the US Presidential election. The coronavirus had little choice but to share its spotlight with Donald Trump and Joe Biden while the world was enraptured by the first world spectacle.

Since the Second World War, the United States has had a role in the world. The president had a responsibility in four key areas: global leadership; defence and promotion of the liberal international order; defence and promotion of freedom, democracy, and human rights; and prevention of the emergence of regional hegemonies in Eurasia.

According to the Congressional Research Service, the traditional role in the world in terms of global leadership means that the United States tends to be the first or most important country for identifying or framing international issues, taking actions to address those issues, setting an example for other countries to follow, organizing and implementing multilateral efforts to address international issues, and enforcing international rules and norms. Hence why the president of the United States or POTUS has always been described as leader of the free world, superpower, indispensable power, system administrator, hyperpower, world policeman, or world hegemon.

> The United States has been described as pursuing an internationalist foreign policy; a foreign policy of global engagement or deep engagement; a foreign policy that provides global public goods; a foreign policy of liberal order building, liberal internationalism,

or liberal hegemony; an interventionist foreign policy; or a foreign policy of seeking primacy or world hegemony.

Reading further into this CRS report, the second key element of the traditional US role in the world since World War II has been to defend and promote the liberal international order including the following:

- Respect for the territorial integrity of countries, and the unacceptability of changing international borders by force or coercion
- A preference for resolving disputes between countries peacefully, without the use or threat of use of force or coercion, and in a manner consistent with international law
- Respect for international law, global rules and norms, and universal values, including human rights
- Strong international institutions for supporting and implementing international law, global rules and norms, and universal values
- The use of liberal international trading and investment systems to advance open, rules-based economic engagement, development, growth, and prosperity
- The treatment of international waters, international air space, outer space, and (more recently) cyberspace as international commons rather than domains subject to national sovereignty

A world class role model. And then there's Donald Trump and his adversary Joe Biden.

Before the pandemic kicked in, Donald John Trump was a 'perceived winner'. Set aside his less than polished demeanour who, unlike Ronald Reagan, was more suited for Hollywood than the White House (he was after all a former reality star) he makes no apologies for his penchant for media notoriety. But under his term America enjoyed its unemployment rate for fifty years. The poorest quarter of workers were growing by 4.7 per cent a year, small-business confidence was near a thirty-year peak, he restricted immigration, brokered peace between Israel and Muslim countries such as the UAE. His campaign slogan 'Make America Great Again' showed his priority to focus on domestic issues than the rest of the world, attributing to his three-pronged strategy of tax cuts, deregulation and confrontational trade policy. As reported in the *Economist*, 'As global economic growth slowed sharply in 2018 and 2019, America's growth fell only relatively gently.' It was not perfect but even economists agreed Trump created a buoyant economy and that was important to America and international business.

But Trump loves friction. He launched a trade war with China and imposed tariffs which hurt and weighed on global growth. And because America (as you realize by now) is a big deal, the IMF estimated that the fight between the two countries might wipe nearly 1 per cent of global output. These were pre-pandemic days.

Trump also had little time for the North Atlantic Treaty Organization (NATO) due to housekeeping matters. Leading up to the election, Trump got infected with the virus, fought over the Supreme Court after the Honourable Ruth Bader Ginsburg passed away, and there was his tax returns disclosure. The region of Nagorno-Karabakh, stuck between the Turkish-supported Azerbaijan and Russia's Armenia, is in dispute. In ten days, 200 soldiers have been killed and increased violence creeping in. A plebiscite has been discussed for decades and thanks to the intervention of Russia and the US, a ceasefire was reached in 1994. With Turkey an ally in NATO this helped to put a lid on things. However, now that both leaders, Trump and Putin, are looking inwards rather than outwards, efforts of peacemaking have slowed to a pace that allows frozen conflicts to turn hot. Until their interest returns, tension persists in conflict regions making them vulnerable to politic-hungry opportunists. This is how seminal the role of POTUS in asserting global peace and policy framing[2].

But that isn't the kind of friction Trump seems interested in. More so now as his position in the White House is on the rocks and the pandemic has challenged the status quo of his previously owned supremacy.[3]

---

[2] By November 2020, thanks to Russia's intervention, Nagorno-Karabakh ceased the fight and agreed to a peace deal and be placed under Russian control. Protesters called for Armenia's prime minister Nikol Pashinyan to resign.

[3] As of the time of this writing i.e. 6 November 2020, ballots are still being counted. Trump may lose his position but the delay in counting the ballots raises his suspicions of fraud. He may not be keen to step down without getting the Supreme court involved, kicking up a media storm and setting the US democracy on fire.

Under his term Trump took many unorthodox approaches. Soon after his swearing-in in 2016 he abandoned the Trans-Pacific Partnership trade talks and signed a Muslim travel ban; in 2017, he withdrew from the Paris agreement on climate change and from the Iran nuclear deal; in 2018 he withdrew from the Intermediate-Range Nuclear Forces Treaty (INF) with Russia and placed a $300 billion import tariffs on Chinese goods; and most notably, withdrew from the World Health Organization (claiming suspicion against China) which placed a major dent in the pandemic race as America is WHO's biggest donor providing around 15 per cent of its budget in 2019. According to the *Economist*, Trump visited the least number of countries. He averaged at twenty-two per year of term compared to George H. W. Bush, Bill Clinton, George W. Bush and Barack Obama at seventy-four each.

Trump is like a cockroach. You can beat him with allegations and flush him with accusations of desecrating the democracy and values of the citizens of the United States but that won't exterminate him. Conversely that might be what strengthens his resilience.

Joseph Robinette Biden Jr served as the forty-seventh vice president of the United States in the Obama administration (2009-2017). People close to Barack Obama's 2008 campaign have said they had real concerns about Biden, most centrally about his ability to stay on message and his propensity for political gaffes. He also has early stages of dementia. Trump has called Biden 'Sleepy Joe' and termed his Democratic opponent just plain 'stupid.' After taking the Montreal Cognitive Assessment (a screening test for dementia), Trump said, 'Joe should take that test, because something's going on . . . We can't have somebody that's not 100 per cent.' Trump isn't entirely wrong.

Trump's son Eric has appeared on Fox News to make a similar point. Biden, he said, 'doesn't have the mental capacity to be Commander-in-chief of this country.' More importantly, true.

There are several known medical issues and risks in Biden's history: his age, his history of a brain aneurysm and repair in 1988, and his reported atrial fibrillation and anticoagulation. Experts have suggested that these issues increase Biden's risk of small, silent strokes.

Would the gravitas of his role if elected as President take a massive toll and precipitate his condition?

And there is also the side agenda. It isn't foreign information that Biden has been a tool for presidential politics. As a contrast to Obama, Biden's appeal among white working-class voters and at a spry sixty-five years old, Obama advisers felt he balanced the age gap between the younger Obama. 'Joe is the pick of my head,' Obama told Tim Kaine, then the governor of Virginia, after he made his choice.

In his run Biden has already made at least one politically strategic choice by limiting the candidates to women. Lisa Lerer from the *New York Times* writes:

> Picking a woman isn't about personal loyalty; it's about energizing female voters and recognizing the momentum that women—particularly Black women—have given the Democratic Party during the Trump era. Given his age, Mr. Biden also needs to reassure voters that there's someone who can take over if he can no longer serve as president—a reason there aren't many older women on the list.

> Criticized as a centrist, an institutionalist, a consensus-builder, the most glaring fact is Biden is too old for the presidential game. Undoubtedly he possesses better public relations skills but winning the election would mean being less the Commander-in-chief the great nation needs but more towards damage control and rebuilding America's decrepit infrastructure starting with repositioning Trump's optics: give more to health and education and allow immigration.

> However, Biden is more human. Unlike Trump, Biden is a pacifist. He listens to experts rather than muzzles them the way Trump did to the Centre of Disease Control, and his vice president is perhaps the reason he will, and needs to, win. Kamala Harris is a Democrat's dream: female, of mixed ethnicity, and the antithesis to Trump's moral bankruptcy. Her win would be at a much needed time even for the Republicans as America grows more diverse. Their strategy is clear; Biden comes

in as the situational leader to put the broken pieces together, and it will be Harris as the transformational leader to synergize the fragments. Harris represents the future. She offers a glimpse to what America should and could become and that's what all political elections are about.

Between conjecture and actualization, that's a different story. Early exit polls on 3 November showed Biden's supporters ticked racial inequality as priority number one. According to CNN, six out of every ten Trump supporters said the economy is their biggest concern. And that's the problem that may win Donald Trump the Presidential election. *Priorities*. If the polls are teaching us anything, it's racial, economic and gender disparity which are wider than realized.

The Issues That Are Motivating 2020 Voters

Share of **Biden voters** and **Trump voters** who said the following issues were "very important" in deciding whom to vote for:

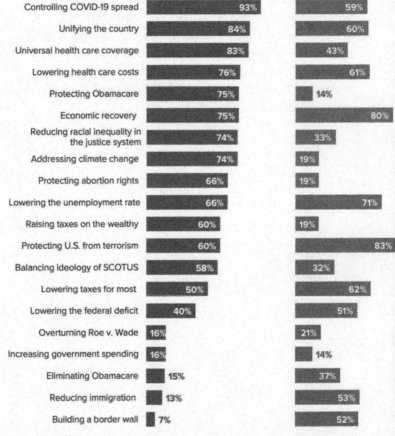

Issue	Biden voters	Trump voters
Controlling COVID-19 spread	93%	59%
Unifying the country	84%	60%
Universal health care coverage	83%	43%
Lowering health care costs	76%	61%
Protecting Obamacare	75%	14%
Economic recovery	75%	80%
Reducing racial inequality in the justice system	74%	33%
Addressing climate change	74%	19%
Protecting abortion rights	66%	19%
Lowering the unemployment rate	66%	71%
Raising taxes on the wealthy	60%	19%
Protecting U.S. from terrorism	60%	83%
Balancing ideology of SCOTUS	58%	32%
Lowering taxes for most	50%	62%
Lowering the federal deficit	40%	51%
Overturning Roe v. Wade	16%	21%
Increasing government spending	16%	14%
Eliminating Obamacare	15%	37%
Reducing immigration	13%	53%
Building a border wall	7%	52%

⊻ MORNING CONSULT

Poll conducted Oct. 30-Nov. 3, 2020, among 11,822 Americans who voted early or on Election Day, with a margin of error of +/-1%.

In an exit poll conducted by CNN on 3 November the key concerns were greatly different. Trump voters were motivated by recovering the economy, tackling terrorism and lowering unemployment rate. Biden supporters were concerned with COVID-19, unifying the country and universal healthcare coverage.

With the slim margin between the two candidates, it all boils down to a slight movement of the needle and electoral college votes. The match point rests on everything else including crime and safety but very little on the obvious i.e. the coronavirus. Seems like the panic is not as dire as projected despite the 234,000 infected rate (as of 4 November 2020). In that sense, Trump's downplaying of the pandemic may prove a point.

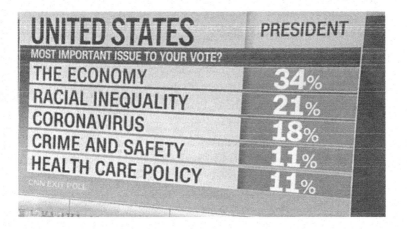

That brings us to the question of priorities as these key concerns will swing the extra voters needed for each candidate.

Counting the votes took time. An uncomfortably long time. Anxiety levels were high throughout the country, even around the world. Twitter and Facebook have been busy round the clock censoring and flagging fake information critical in skewering public opinion especially in the weeks leading up to the election. This was a pivotal moment as we were witnessing a nation known for being a military, economic and cultural superpower, fighting itself between two factions. It felt like a yard fight between two populists: one, a nasty politician and another, an ageing centrist. The media too became questionable in terms of being honest, valid and reliable with their reporting. There were flip states, sudden surge of votes, suspicious delay of counting the votes and anxiety over Sharpie pens invalidating votes, suddenly people begged the question: was this the US presidential election or a third world-level political election? And on the moral front it was obvious at this juncture that the vote was less on selecting the next leader of the free world but more to garner enough votes to get rid of its existing president. Celebrities turned to their social media expressing their sentiments on the candidates. Was social media doing a disservice to them by rubbing salt to wounds and heightening anxiety to sway, irate and manipulate sentiments? This raises a new lesson for future campaigns. President Trump continued to question the legitimacy of the vote count in subsequent Twitter posts, some of which have been blocked by the social media platform and threatened to take legal action.

Former Democrat presidential contender Bernie Sanders made an appearance on *The Tonight Show* with Jimmy Fallon on October 23, during which he predicted how the delay in counting pre-poll votes would set President Trump off in a bid to prematurely claim victory in the US election. And he was correct.

President Trump held a press conference in the White House just after 2 a.m. local time on 4 November, at which he claimed victory. He claimed the poll had been subject to 'fraud'.

> 'Frankly, we did win this election,' President Trump said. 'So our goal now is to ensure integrity, for the good of this nation—this is a very big moment, this is a major fraud on our nation. We want the law to be used in a proper manner, so we'll be going to the US Supreme Court. We want all voting to stop. We don't want them to find any ballots at 4 o'clock in the morning and add them to the list. It's a very sad moment.

5 November the counting dragged on. According to exit polling, nine in ten Biden voters and 84 per cent of Trump voters agreed with the sentiment that it's time to wrap up the contest, producing the smallest

gap between the two sets of supporters among the feelings tested in the poll.

Meanwhile the world waits in bated breath.

But why was the entire US presidential election rigmarole so seminal to the rest of the world?

History tells us that leaders come out at times where they're tested and tried. Despite its flaws, failings and supposedly fading dominance, America is still seen as an emotional and moral benchmark internationally. In almost every mainstream and popular culture, America has come to be this omnipresent character that constantly reinvents itself and bounces back from very problematic circumstances.

Everything about the United States is mighty. According to NBCNews.com, the United States spent $732 billion on its military in 2019, almost three times that of second place China. It has around 5,800 nuclear warheads, and the United States' gross domestic product of more than $20 trillion still outstrips that of Beijing or the European Union. Journalist Alexander Smith writes, 'Part of the explanation, so the theory goes, is that many people outside the US maintain a deep, emotional investment, consciously or otherwise, in America's founding mythos: a flawed work-in-progress that nonetheless has the potential to fulfil its founding aspirations of democracy, liberty and equality.'

'There's still this sense that stuff that happens in America matters to all of us,' Adam Smith, a professor of US politics and history at the University of Oxford, said. 'Because if they screw it up, then we're really screwed.'

In 1835, the French diplomat Alexis de Tocqueville published *Democracy in America,* a book based on his travels to the New World where he observed its attempts to build a democracy on the nascent values of the Enlightenment. The Enlightenment, also known as the Age of Reason, was an intellectual and cultural movement in the eighteenth century that emphasized reason over superstition and science over blind faith. Many countries on the cusp of its independence looked to the Enlightenment as a paradigm for its constitutional foundation.

And with Donald Trump, it's a cautionary tale for leadership studies, starting with how *not* to be an execrated leader.

But it's also an interesting study of how the US came to this predicament. After all, Trump did not place himself in the White House. He was voted there. And if he feels a concern to remain in the White House in order to protect Americans' rights and constitution, that is his exertion of the First Amendment as a citizen and Commander-in-chief, one of the ten amendments that constitute the Bill of Rights 1791.

The US has set high moral standards for itself through documents and speeches such as the Declaration of Independence, the Gettysburg Address, and President Woodrow Wilson's '14 points' (a statement of principles for peace that was to be used for peace negotiations in order to end World War I) that set out a model for peace in postwar Europe so when we see those standards slip with President Donald Trump's rhetorical tone, endemic racism and his coronavirus response, there is a great binary of disappointment and exciting hope that the nation can overcome this.

But Trumpwatching is not just a global love affair with America. Citizens the world over are obsessed with their own leaders and it has been one of the oldest sports. We have an insatiable desire to read about what they say and do, watch them, rate them, and pass judgment on them. And with social media, the flood of comments lies at the heart of the nation's conversation.

According to Jeff Kehoe of *Harvard Business Review Press*, the mania is not really on figureheads but on us:

> While the mutual obsession between us and our presidents will no doubt continue—the onslaught of communications, whether mediated or not, will only intensify as digital platforms gain power—it's important to remember that, ultimately, it is we citizens who determine our political leaders' fate and legacy. Lincoln once said: 'Public sentiment is everything. With public sentiment, nothing can fail; without it, nothing can succeed.' He was right. When presidents communicate, well or badly, our response is what matters. We are the ones in charge.

Maybe it's because our culture only understands hierarchy.

According to historian Thomas Carlyle a leader is 'one gifted with unique qualities that capture the imagination of the masses.'

Traditionally, people believed that leaders were born with the natural gift to lead. Known as the Great Man theory Odysseus, Ashoka, Alexander the Great were figures bestowed with strength believed to be by divinity and guided by seers. They were The Chosen One. They were looked up as Gods and were the rule of law. No one dared to question their decisions and their soldiers marched into battles willing to die for them. As time went by people realized that great leaders were developed not born. With every passing war and catastrophic event, leaders were gradually seen as courageous mortals with exceptional skills for communication and strategy. The fact that they were human and not demigods made them relatable but positioned at the top of the social hierarchy.

The presence of wars created a convenient canvas for leaders like Winston Churchill, Napoleon Bonaparte and Franklin D. Roosevelt to demonstrate their fortitude. These leaders were the embodiment of the saying that 'The pen is mightier than the sword'. Unlike their predecessors who proved physical strength at the battlefield and were born into their role, the modern leaders were elected by the people and were role models as thinkers, arbitrators and negotiators. A few, however, took their trusted authority a few steps too far.

Adolf Hitler, Joseph Stalin and Mao Zedong taught us that leaders too can abuse power. But a leader gathers no strength without loyal subjects, and to be a great leader you need great adversaries which is why audiences love Marvel and DC heroes. The model is: the more illustrious the enemies, the greater the challenges, the more outstanding the hero is perceived.

Collective consciousness: The Batman mythology

Carl Jung and Joseph Campbell looked at how archetypes, universal themes we inherit as part of our collective unconscious, symbolically shape myths and legends of heroes in similar ways throughout every culture in the world. According to them, the so-called 'Hero's Journey' represents individuals' own psychological growth as they confront features of their personal and collective unconscious in order to grow, mature, and fulfil their potential as human beings. The shadow archetype represents your own dark side, the part of you that is hidden, out of the light, the sum of those characteristics you conceal from both the world and yourself. Bruce Wayne confronts his own darkest nature early in life, chooses to work with it, and uses it to instil fear in others. His bright and dark sides work together to fight evil. From a Jungian perspective, therefore, Batman appeals to our own need to face and manage our own shadow selves. We want Batman in our shadows.

In the History Channel documentary *Batman Unmasked: The Psychology of the Dark Knight,* the masked crusader, a fictional character created by Bob Kane and introduced in *Detective Comics #27* in 1939, is Bruce Wayne, a man who witnessed his parents gunned down as a young boy and was adopted and raised by altruistic parents who taught him to help those who have less than himself. He suffers a phobia for bats and what makes Wayne a popular and most analysed hero by psychologists and psychiatrists is his human vulnerability that represents the potential hero in all of us.

With the inherited fortune from his affluent parents, Wayne creates Batman, his alter ego who fights crime and dedicates his life to creating justice in the dark, crime-ridden city of Gotham. Wayne selects Batman as a way to face his chiroptophobia and self-imposes combating crime as a way to vindicate his biological parents' death. There have been more movies spawned by understanding Batman's personal journey (the *Dark Knight* franchise) in recent years compared to Superman and Spiderman; audiences begin to move away from demigods such as Superman and freaked heroes like Spiderman (bitten by a radioactive spider) for human resonance and interconnectedness.

However, Batman has no story without his supervillains. And he has thirty-seven of them.

Psychoanalysts point out that Batman and his enemies have a common thread: all are victims of personal or childhood trauma and PTSD. The difference however, is that Batman consciously chooses to face his childhood wounds to positive advantage while his enemies succumb to theirs. Wayne transforms his biggest fear to become his formidable strength while his enemies channel theirs as vengeance to punish the world. Mired in their personal pain, Two-Face, Scarecrow, Solomon Grundy, and frequently encountered archenemy The Joker to name a few were unfortunate individuals mistreated and untimely violated before turning evil that we find ourselves feeling for them as much as supporting Batman. The turn of the screw became increasingly evident as more spin-offs began to portray backstories of notable villains, such as *Maleficent* (from *Sleeping Beauty*) and *Joker*.

The insurgence of superhero movies is a sign of the times, we are in need of leaders to look up to. More importantly, citizens today are in need to *feel* their leaders. Gradually we move further away from the perfect hero imagery. Daniel Craig's outing of James Bond has Agent 007 as someone who not only bleeds but sheds tears and suffers from heartbreak. Mal Vincent of the *Virginian-Pilot* writes, '(In *Casino Royale*), Bond is grieving over the death of Vesper and is wondering if she had betrayed him to boot. He learns that she didn't actually do him wrong; it was the bad guys who made her do it. He loved her.'

Coincidentally on Halloween, Sean Connery passed away. The world mourns the original James Bond who, unlike Craig's portrayal, was the quintessential agent. Connery's death signifies a kairotic moment where heroes are now far from perfect. He was becoming flawed and familiar.

This explains why Donald Trump, vile and racist as he is, remained strong in the 2020 US presidential race. **Is it the vote or the voice that counts?** The over-performance of his poll numbers everywhere proved he was not losing this election easily to Biden as many thought. According to CNN's report:

> Whether President Donald Trump ultimately wins or loses a second term, Tuesday's election proved something beyond the shadow of a doubt: He has broken modern politics. Or, to put a finer point on it: Trump has exposed the way we poll, analyse and predict election outcomes.
>
> Heading into Election Day, every shred of available evidence suggested that Trump was likely to lose, and lose convincingly, to former Vice President Joe Biden. The incumbent trailed by high single-digits in national polling. He was behind in polling averages in virtually every swing state. He was being drastically outspent on television in the vast majority of battlegrounds. Professional campaign handicappers were unanimous: This election was likely to border on landslide territory for Biden.
>
> And yet, that's not what happened. While you'd almost certainly rather be Biden than Trump at this point when you look at where votes remain to be counted in critical swing states like Wisconsin, Michigan and Pennsylvania, it's clear that the incumbent, if he loses, will not be swept out of office in a clear rebuke of his first four years in office.

America experienced the most number of voters since 1900. Florida and Texas, despite their diversity, shifted towards the Republicans. Though Trump dogwhistles about immigrants and makes derogatory comments about women, he won the Latino votes in the sunny states, presenting to us a cautionary tale about minorities being monolithic. The political divide also shows a problem that looms ahead for America even if Biden wins: America today is a nation diverse and a nation divided. To repudiate Trump and his Trumponomics is to downplay the voices of the greater Americans and to ignore the fact that almost half of the population felt Trump was suited to remain as President of the United States. He may not be the perfect hero portrayed in Hollywood staples or rise from the ashes like President Kirkman in *Designated Survivor*, but he spoke of truths over idealisms.

In a letter to the Editor of *Fillmore County Journal*, a reader Gerald J. Boyum of Rochester, Minnesota, posts (18 March 2020):

> As expected, the leftist media is exploiting the COVID-19 pandemic to smear him (Trump) as a complete 'failure' and even describing him as a 'sociopath' while gleefully discussing how this pandemic can help the Democratic Socialists in 2020.
>
> Why do Leftists hate America? America is a massive refutation of their utopian fantasy, universal equality. They compare America with their vision of a perfect country which has never existed. Rather than change their false theories, they lash out at America and conservatives, including Trump.
>
> If we consider a 'perfect' country, it is not hard to find problems in America: racial prejudice, economic exploitation and inequality, greed, etc. However, countries do not exist in fantasyland; they exist in the real world. However, the world that surrounds us is not too idyllic. If we compare the US to its surroundings, America is the one that begins to resemble an idealized paradise. Otherwise, why do so many foreign nationals risk life and limb to get to America?

In any election, the overriding consideration in voting should be the political ideologies associated with candidates and the direction America should take. Is it:

a. American Conservatism, promoted by Republicans and founded on Biblical/Christian principles that have resulted in the greatest country to have ever existed? Or,

b. Democratic Socialism, based on godless Marxism that has resulted in catastrophic failure with over 100 million people murdered by their governments in the 20th century alone, with millions more living in poverty and misery whenever and wherever it's been tried?

This is one of the many Republican voices of America, and Trump speaks this language fluently. All over the world there are countries ruled by political leaders who stand between promising idealism and demystifying them. With the domination of social media and memes, people today have grown accustomed to obnoxious figureheads who say it like it is. The modern American voters now stand between those who believe in the Superman leader and those who believe in an imperfect mortal. While the imperfect hero will continuously be criticised for making mistakes (it happened to the charming Obamas too), the Superman leader will face mounting pressure to live up to high expectations and to continuously play with the imagery of the idealised American dream.

As for the Democrats, a flaw in their idealised system lies in the fact that the population for the non-educated Americans remains high (36 per cent of Americans have a bachelor's degree) and the constitutional rhetoric and multilateral economic policies are spoken by the upper bracket and privileged liberals. To them Trump is uncouth. Yet Trump managed to swing votes from non-college, young African and Hispanic voters. As for the Democrats, even if Biden wins, they failed to secure power in the senate meaning the Biden-Harris agenda will be an uphill climb. According to the reports, Republicans have sharply cut Democrats' chances of taking back the Senate, winning a series of contests across the country on the coattails of President Trump. At this point, the future stewardship of America regardless who wins, needs to focus on regaining not so much the American voice, but more critically, a united voice. The bitter truth remains that polarized societies place a great strain on democracy. And this may not be the last of Trumpism. There's also the presidential election in 2024.

For now, according to the Political Intelligence US exit polls as of 6 November at 5.23 p.m. Malaysian time, voters on both sides resoundingly agree on one thing: they just want this election to be over.

Postscript: As of 8.05 a.m. on Sunday 8 November 2020 Biden has won the election. The question for Trump by the people: Will he step down peacefully? The question for Biden by governments everywhere: How will America affect their national interest? As they say in Japan, *ganbatte kudasai*, which stands for 'please do your best' or 'keep it up' or 'I know you can do it' depending on the situation. In this case for America and its next president, it applies for all three.

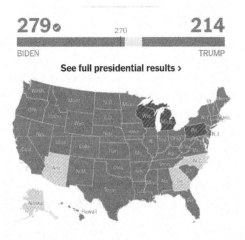

The New York Times

BIDEN BEATS TRUMP

Harris Is First Woman Elected Vice President

279 ⊘   270   **214**

BIDEN   TRUMP

See full presidential results ›

Mental Housekeeping

'He is no hero who never met the dragon.'
Carl Jung

'The returning hero, to complete his adventure, must survive the impact of the world.'
Joseph Campbell

The coronavirus has upended our lives to levels that even experts are forced to relearn our coping mechanism. Capsized travel plans, panic over scarce resources and information overload could be a recipe for unchecked anxiety and feelings of isolation. However, it is indefinite isolation that becomes the subject of concern.

While isolation isn't new to us, the trigger is in the newness of the phenomena: indefinite timelines, a novel virus outbreak, new vaccines, new norms, governmental restructuring, even new leaders. According to American mythologist, writer and lecturer Joseph Campbell, moments like these are necessary turning points of our lives. 'Opportunities to find deeper powers within ourselves come when life seems most challenging.' Through his book *The Hero With a Thousand Faces* published in 1949, Campbell believed that intense hardships are what build us and enrich our lives in the pursuit of 'the Hero's journey', an archetypal rite of passage we cannot avoid. The Hero's Journey provides us with a mythical lens where one has to endure three phases in order to fully claim himself victorious: call to adventure, ordeal, victory. In between these phases are many decisions and crossroads embroiled in fear, suffering, struggle. Campbell writes, 'A hero ventures forth from the world of common day into a region of supernatural wonder: fabulous forces are encountered there and a decisive victory is won: the hero comes back from this mysterious adventure with the power to bestow boons on his fellow man.'

But the transformational mono-myth—especially when applied to the realities of our current situation—is far more labyrinthine. The fabric of our lives is filled with layers of social constructs and limitations that make us fight within ourselves that we often lose sight of the Hero's Journey. As we become more jaded and cynical we elude the journey altogether. What happens then?

'Our bodies and our brains are set up to deal with short-term crises that have clear ends in sight,' says Allison Buskirk-Cohen, associate professor and chair of the psychology department at Delaware Valley University. 'Long-term ambiguous stressors—like managing the COVID-19 situation—are much more challenging.'

According to mental health clinicians, one way to tackle the situation is by doing constant check-ins with yourself. And in the light of the corona, because tomorrow remains unclear, today is what counts. Though we can ask ourselves many questions, the ones on pages 100 and 101 target areas that may likely seem uncomfortable and that's the whole point.

Groundhog day

The 1993 film *Groundhog Day* makes a perfect allegory. Starring Bill Murray and Andie MacDowell the story is similar to *A Christmas Carol* by Charles Dickens, in which Ebenezer Scrooge is visited by ghosts that represent three chapters of his miserable life: past, present and future. With each visit Scrooge gets a reflection of his true character and how the decisions he makes affect others to be just as miserable. This in turn inspires him to become a kind man. In *Groundhog Day* the protagonist Phil is stuck in a repetition of a single day like a supernatural intervention. Phil was nasty, narcissistic and selfish. Forced to wake up to the same day however, made him realize the butterfly effect. Intensely stressful at first, Phil grew to understand how good begets good and vice versa, and if he were to be stuck in an eternal cycle, he could at least create a better existence for himself and others. In short, Phil learns to think of others instead of himself and that is the golden rule. Changing his perception after running out of ways to escape life, Phil stops seeing his predicament as a curse. Rather, he's given a gift of having to repeat the same day over and over until he discovers his purpose.

The time loop may be supernatural, but it serves as a metaphor for a typical life. Many people can relate to Phil's predicament. They feel trapped in the routine of jobs they don't particularly like. They have trouble connecting with others on a deep level. They function OK, but they're profoundly unhappy.

Phil gains knowledge from each passing day, but to everyone else it's as if the previous days never happened. At a closer inspection, Phil unwittingly develops a strategy. At first, he deals with his boredom and angst in hedonistic ways. He succumbs to several of the seven deadly sins, including gluttony and sloth. He's shown watching 'Jeopardy!' with other guests at the bed-and-breakfast where he's staying, chugging Jack Daniels and impressing them with trivial knowledge. He begins to think he's immortal. He commits suicide, several times over: by standing in front of a truck, electrocuting himself in a bathtub and diving off a building. Still, he wakes up the next day. 'I am a god,' he says. Phil realizes his own mortality when he discovers an old bum has died.

Transformation begins when Phil starts to take an interest in other people's lives. He takes up new hobbies like ice sculpturing and learns to play the piano. He discovers money will never be a problem after robbing an armoured car, and knowing he can get away with it, uses the cash to improve the lives of the community.

From his new set of skills he develops a heightened appreciation for life. With every improvement, he gains strength to get out of depression, and his interest for Rita, who used to repeatedly slap his face, changes from lust to genuine affection. But it was his gestures towards helping others that finally gave him the true meaning of his existence. He felt purposeful. He grew to become the most beloved person in town and one day, Phil wakes up to a new day; the curse of time has been broken. He has crossed over to victory.

Groundhog Day is not just about the Hero's Journey. American psychologist Carol Dweck would describe Phil's experience to a growth mindset.

Growth mindset

Growth mindset is often mistaken by educators as putting in more hard work. The process according to Dweck is a lot more serpentine. Its basis is that talents and abilities could be developed and that challenges are the way to do it.

> Learning something new, something hard, sticking to things—that's how you get smarter. Setbacks and feedback weren't about your abilities, they were information you could use to help yourself learn. With a growth mindset, we don't necessarily think that there's no such thing as talent or that everyone is the same, but they believe everyone can develop their abilities through hard work, strategies, and lots of help and mentoring from others.
> Carol Dweck, the *Atlantic,* 2016

Dweck describes this effort-based learning as a core component to understanding growth mindset. When students hit a brick wall or procrastinate, instinct is to feel frustrated and defensive. 'Praise the effort that led to the outcome or learning progress; tie the praise to it. It's not just effort, but strategy ... so support the student in finding another strategy.'

Andrew Huberman offers a different interpretation. Huberman calls this DOP—duration, path and outcome—critical in understanding why we procrastinate with anxiety and why procrastination is essential for our growth mindset.

Huberman is a neuroscientist and tenured Professor in the Department of Neurobiology at the Stanford University School of Medicine. His contributions include modern understanding in fields of brain development, brain function and neural plasticity, which is the ability of our nervous system to rewire and learn new behaviours, skills and cognitive functioning.

Huberman is also actively involved in developing tools used by elite military in the US and Canada, athletes, and technology industries for optimizing performance in high stress environments, enhancing neural plasticity, mitigating stress, and optimizing sleep.

Huberman, a colleague of Dweck, was in a podcast interview with Rich Roll discussing neuroplasticity and ways in which the brain shifts our thought patterns. At one point in the interview, Roll shared a problem he was facing: 'Why is it that a person can take weeks to procrastinate an important task but once you really sit down to work on it, that is all you can think about?'

Huberman explains, 'On a daily basis the brain is wired to operate based on a reflex. The way we react and respond to our environment is based on a composite of hardwiring which we accumulate from the ages of 0-25. By then we are cooked in our ways and the quality of data we input determines the quality of output through our thoughts and behaviors.'

In *Focus: The Hidden Driver of Excellence* Daniel Goleman points out a unique discovery regarding procrastination in various settings.

> The longer someone ignores an email before finally responding, the more relative social power that person has. Map these response times across an entire organization and you get a remarkably accurate chart of the actual social standing. The boss leaves emails unanswered for hours or days; those lower down respond within minutes. There's an algorithm for this, a data mining method called 'automated social hierarchy detection,' developed at Columbia University. When applied to the archive of email traffic at Enron Corporation before it folded, the method correctly identified the roles of top-level managers and their subordinates just by how long it took them to answer a given person's emails. Intelligence agencies have been applying the same metric to suspected terrorist gangs, piecing together the chain of influence to spot the central figures.

Huberman's theory is that a lot of how we react and respond to things is based on social conditioning stemming from our upbringing. In short, that's all we know and we tend to adhere to the familiar because it gives us a sense of security, even if deep down it makes us unhappy and we know some of the teachings may be damaging. This leads us to experience the same feedback from our surroundings. This includes attracting the same people, predictable situations and repeating ideas and decisions. Experts call this hardwiring and it blocks new opportunities from coming in. It's difficult to experience growth when you're not challenged with new circumstances. Thus, we need to undo the hardwiring. Rebuild. As Alfred Kotter describes, 'Learn, then unlearn and relearn.'

However, when we attempt a new event the brain needs to warm up, to hone up the circuits, and when that happens, it will not feel comfortable. Fight-or-flight instinct kicks in. The trick to success lies in a combination of the following: You choose fight, develop willpower to soldier through and understand the changes happening; hone the discomfort to help you develop sharper focus on what you're attempting; allow the stress and confusion to transform into a positive feeling which consequently helps you to be good at acquiring new skill.

The early stages of hard work and focus will naturally feel like a combination of agitation, stress and confusion. And that's what's needed in order to get your brain to find the right circuits to do a few things: Understand what's happening and the challenges involved. Norepinephrine and your entire adrenaline system are kicking in, funnelling into the groove of this new circuitry.

Dopamine works with your nervous system to send messages between nerve cells to say something significant is happening and that positive energy triggers an internal reward system which explains why and how you become increasingly good at the task at hand. Dopamine plays a role in how we feel pleasure which becomes part of the intrinsic reward. It's a big part of our unique human ability to think and plan.

Thanks to movies like *Groundhog Day* we can better understand the corona matrix we are in. However the profound truth is that it doesn't take a virus or a supernatural intervention to push us to realize our

Hero's Journey. But now that we are here, we can begin to take hold of our transformation.

Embracing the struggles by gestures and communication can help to peter out the anxiety we accrue from the mundane and repetitive days. Intra-communication (engagement within oneself) is more crucial than inter-personal (engaging with others).

Self-directed introspection, says experts, is as important as deep breathing exercises. Not only are you giving yourself space to think, but you also have the power to alter how you think. Because what you tell yourself is exactly what you digest, penning your thoughts takes you closer to affirmation and goal-setting. Most importantly, self check-ins help to induce or reignite dormant creativity and curiosity, allowing you a chance to rediscover and reconnect with yourself. In some cases, this goes as far back as your childhood. There is research to suggest a correlation between childhood teasings to anxieties in adulthood, and isolation caused by the lockdown can trigger latent traumas. As lockdown increases isolation for many, this also ceases communication. People living alone, being displaced or separated by their loved ones can develop generalised anxiety disorder (GAD).

Here's a journal exercise you can do at your own comfortable pace. The key is to deep dive into each question without a word limit. Each question can be attempted at different times to observe your underlying thoughts.

Twenty questions to ask yourself during lockdown

What should be the goal for these self check-ins? A chance for answers that can lead to a new sense of discovery. By the time the corona curtains are uplifted you have new paths to venture forth. To quote the great Sir Ken Robinson who died on 21 August 2020, 'Life is not linear. When you follow your own true north you create new opportunities, meet different people, have different experiences and create a different life.'

Once out of this lockdown there will be no better time presented to us to really focus on our inner healing. Time, in all manners, is a gift. These questions are designed to help you begin your Hero's Journey. Bon voyage.

1. How is my body feeling?
2. What emotions am I feeling?
3. Am I being too hard on myself?
4. Am I expecting too much from others?
5. What is bothering me? Is it important?
6. What new habits do I want to form right now?
7. What do I want to learn from this experience/event?
8. What have I been procrastinating?
9. Who am I agitated with?
10. How am I spending my time on social media?
11. Have I read anything useful?
12. What seems to be a useless waste of time?
13. Have I had a meaningful conversation?
14. Have I formed new friendships recently?

15. Am I losing/renewing interest in my job?
16. Have I been recalling my childhood?
17. What do I miss about my childhood?
18. Who do I miss the most? Write a letter you don't intend to send.
19. Do I have beef with anyone I wish I could reconcile with? Write a heartfelt letter to say how you feel or to apologize for your half.
20. Have I planned my new life? Imagine being sent to prison for a crime you did commit. You will be up for parole soon. Here's your chance for atonement with yourself.

Staying Sane in a time of insanity

'The 3 Cs in life:
Choice, Chance, Change.
You must make the choice,
To take the chance,
If you want anything
in life to change.'
@healdocumentary

This may sound absurd, but chaos can be a good reset button and a call to action. It pushes you out of a reverie, exercises our senses and hammers the snooze button we have been pressing incessantly. One way to massage our creativity during a quarantine is to reimagine the life you want to live, the person you want to be, the relationships you want to rebuild or to reconcile when the dust settles. Close your eyes and think: *How do you visualise yourself coming out of this long, dark tunnel?* Aged, haggard and bitter? Taller, better adapted to life and glowing? You describe.

Next we come to the heart of our darkness. *Who do we become* and *who have we become* since we fell into the clutches of corona? Social experts would say how we respond and react to situations reveal the core of our inner wounds, the childhood traumas that have yet to be healed. Why is it that we seem to stay connected through our gadgets yet when faced with actual family time with no options, we seem to fray at the seams?

Have I been living a restless lie? Many would realize at this point how their life has been on auto-pilot. For many businesses, working from home will uplift the veil to show that being at the office is, and should be, optional. And now faced with having to conduct real conversations in confined spaces with their significant other or loved ones, new realities emerge; how do we begin a meaningful conversation? Have you forgotten how it feels?

In an interview with athlete-turned-show host of *The School of Greatness* Lewis Howes, author and psychotherapist Esther Perel provides a good case study: Two firefighter pilots who fought in Iraq and Afghanistan set up a successful company together. Then one decides to leave the other threatening to rock the foundation of the company. Conflicted at a junction, two questions were raised for them to reflect: Were we successful because we had a great idea? Or were we successful because we had each other? This creates a perfect matrix to place every relationship out there that is swinging over a burning pit. Or at least by day twelve that is how it feels.

The life we've created, do we like it? Viktor Frankl in his book, *Man's Search For Meaning*, questions how we validate our existence through our relationships and experiences. He develops the theory of logotherapy and describes, 'You cannot change your circumstances, but you can change your response to the circumstances, and that you have, until the very last moment, the fundamental freedom, which is the meaning that you give to what is happening around you.' Frankl survived the Holocaust and writes from this context, using the power of creativity through narratives.

He chronicled his experiences in a tiny notebook and at one point when he lost it, questioned if his entire existence had any meaning without a body of proof. But the marvel of Frankl's work was in identifying a purpose in life to feel positive about, and then immersively imagining that outcome. In short, it is what lies ahead that motivates your survival. Many cancer patients will tell you they fought to stay alive for their children and loved ones. They focused on goals and imagined running towards the finishing line as they fought the effects of surgery, chemo and radiation therapy.

Resting upon the existential doctrine of Kierkegaard's 'will to meaning', Frankl's work is relevant to us today as we redefine the meaning of our lives while being held in isolation and in restriction.

This is a good time to ask ourselves, what motivates us in our life? What is the driving force? Perhaps this was the Pandora's box that opened for the people in China. The government lockdown, the scarcity of resources and near death experience shocked them to reimagine life with a blessed second chance, and a divorce is perhaps seen as just a small price to pay for a greater meaning to life. Bickering over house chores was just a simpler reason over the existential dilemma.

Frankl identifies three psychological reactions experienced by all inmates to one degree or another which can be used as a COVID quarantine model: one, shock during the initial admission phase to the isolation or lockdown, two, apathy after becoming accustomed, especially if governments prolong the duration, and three, reactions of depersonalization, moral deformity, bitterness, and disillusionment when we are liberated.

Whatever that lies ahead should matter less if we are mentally, emotionally and physically prepared. My two takeaways on how to stay balanced during the MCO or a lockdown would be as follows.

Have a structure. Design your daily routine. Just as every meeting must establish its objectives and intended outcome, wake up with a set of goals to accomplish rather than worry about what is going to happen. It doesn't mean you are restricted from allowing your day to flow organically but a structure provides a deeper meaning to what you are doing, and when you achieve a task, there is a sense of achievement. Structure conversations the same way to avoid meandering towards petty arguments and finger pointing.

In the event an argument ensues, take a step back to ask yourself three questions: One, why am I upset? Two, what triggered me? Three, is it *who* or is it *what made* me upset? Do not attempt to discuss until you have these three figured out. Apologizing is polishing half the truth, and that does not remove the splinter that caused the argument.

Gain perspective. Accept what you can and let go of what you can't. In 2006 I experienced severe blizzards in Minnesota, United States. The weather had turned so drastically it was declared Emergency. Town folks couldn't leave the house or you will freeze to death. Temperature plummeted to minus forty-eight degrees Celsius. It was there I realized that Mother Nature has an erratic mind of her own. You can go out in the heat of summer at ninety-two degrees Celsius and suddenly without warning the temperature can drop to thirty-eight degrees. For the first time I was experiencing snow storms with my house covered in twelve feet of snow. I was locked in up to eight days with no sun, saw no people, had no TV or the internet. It was just grey days and lots of coffee, no appetite. Seeing another human walk down the street was all I needed to comfort me, to know I was not alone. My town folks did exactly what happened in China. We stayed in and we stayed occupied and fed with whatever means we had. This changes perspectives. Once the weather cleared and life was back to normal, I spoke to neighbours who had lived in the area for decades. Here they taught me a valuable lesson on perspective: in life, things happen. You can either see it as a disaster or you can see it as an experience. You have that choice. But things will happen. You just become better at knowing what to do when it does.

COVID-19 is the invisible snowstorm that has locked us in our own psychological and sociological spheres. This is perhaps the Universe's satirical gift to mankind. We are restless, we are uncertain, and we have yet to fully grasp the aftermath. But this compromising condition is what allows us to move towards growth.

Perhaps it was time to lose that last 6 kg. Perhaps it was time to admit the intimacy is gone. Perhaps it's time you took that job and finished that 5000 piece jigsaw puzzle. Perhaps it was time you faced your difficult mother and listened without prejudice. Perhaps it was time you hugged your panic-stricken sibling instead of telling her to calm down. Perhaps COVID-19 is teaching us to listen more, to feel more, to forgive more and to simply let go.

And like the snowstorms in Minnesota, eventually the sun will come out, the snow will melt and rinse the fuckeries of our past. You will have survived and you will be transformed.

Of life and death

'PETALING JAYA (THE STAR/ASIA NEWS NETWORK): Healthcare workers in Malaysia who were infected with COVID-19 after being vaccinated reported less severe symptoms, said health director-general Noor Hisham Abdullah, even as he cautioned that people who have been vaccinated can still get infected. 'It is clear that we still can be infected after the completion of vaccination but perhaps less in severity,' he said. He added that 40 healthcare workers have been infected with COVID-19 despite being fully vaccinated.' Reported from The *News Straits Times* Malaysia, 19 April 2021

With the vaccine rollout throughout many developed countries, ironically however, the infection rate has shown another uptick. Seems like another circus came to town.

An article by John Berthelsen for the *Asia Sentinel* reads:

Malaysia, which early on in the fight against the COVID-19 coronavirus was one of Asia's leaders, has begun to slip back, with at least some vaccine procurement seemingly diffused among competing parties thought to be aligned with top politicians, ostensibly illegal shots for royalty, low signup rates due to fears of blood clots, and sharply rising new cases.

Malaysia isn't the only one in Southeast Asia, although Malaysia may be the only one behaving like a bull in a china shop in the Asian basin due to too many incompetent (and exorbitantly overpaid) leaders in its cabinet.

The vaccine rollout has opened a new can of worms: vaccine purchase freelancers. Berthelson continues, 'One of the biggest concerns being spoken of in hushed tones within top political circles is that too many interests are freelancing vaccine purchases. Although there has been no confirmation, sources in Kuala Lumpur say Hamzah Zainuddin, the home affairs minister, and Health Minister Adham Baba are among them.'

I sat across the table over high tea with a friend who was keen to get involved. A housewife, she thought it was a good opportunity to make money. She had good reason: her mother was undergoing expensive treatment for stage 4 cancer and required facilitation up to RM20,000 each week. In such hard times it wasn't the logic but the desperation that spoke louder. My advice was to back off. It wasn't optimistic advice to hear. But I am not here to judge. This was the time of corona. We are not the same people prior to March 2020.

Nell was also the friend who was generous and overly concerned with the state of the world. 'What can we do?' she often asked. Perhaps it was the restriction of mobility that made her anxious to constantly want to reach out and affect the world. Goleman offers a rationale.

> We have a bit of self-interest in relieving the misery of others. One school of modern economic theory, following Hobbes, argues that people give to charities in part because of the pleasure they get from imagining either the relief of those they benefit or their own relief from alleviating their sympathetic distress.

This, I thought, made a lot of sense to the flood of donations and volunteerism during the crisis.

Shark in shallow waters

Imagine being held against our will for vaccination. We are armed with so-called trust by the government that is blatantly being reported in the dailies for being corrupt and incompetent (remember the Doraemon advice?).

In a country with a population of over 31.95 million, only a total of 8,602,156 people had registered for the vaccine as of Monday (19 April 2021) through the *MySejahtera*, the national application. That's another display of high-level distrust. In contrast, Israel, Bhutan, and Singapore have reportedly vaccinated at least 28.5 per cent of its citizens. Population may differ but efficiency is distinct.

According to Science, Technology and Innovation Minister Khairy Jamaluddin, who is also the coordinating minister for the National COVID-19 Immunisation Programme, eighty per cent of Malaysians will have received their COVID-19 vaccinations by year's end. From June, he adds, vaccine supply will begin to outstrip the number of registrations for inoculation. By October, he pledges, Malaysia will have enough vaccines for 80 per cent of the population.

As reported in the *New Straits Times*:

The country has just completed phase one of the vaccine programme, which ran from February to April, for front-liners.

The second phase - which will prioritise the elderly, those with comorbidity problems and people with disabilities - will start on April 19.

The third phase of the programme will take place in May for low-risk individuals.

Unfortunately, according to numerous reports like this one in *Medscape* (16 April 2021) by Brenda Goodman, it's a tightrope walk and a juggle of knives.

This is the tentative schedule by the Ministry. At the same time we have these updates riding against the timelines:

> Health director-general Noor Hisham Abdullah cautions that people who have been vaccinated can still get infected. 'It is clear that we still can be infected after the completion of vaccination but perhaps less in severity,' he said. He added that 40 healthcare workers have been infected with COVID-19 despite being fully vaccinated.

On vaccinations, Dr Noor Hisham said that no one is safe until everyone is safe and advised everyone to continue complying with all the precautionary public health measures.

New evidence emerged today tying vaccines for COVID-19 to extremely rare cases of people who develop blood clots and low platelets within weeks of being vaccinated.

A team of researchers in the United Kingdom conducted an in-depth investigation of 22 patients who developed serious blood clots combined with a drop in blood platelets after receiving a dose of the AstraZeneca vaccine, which is now called Vaxzevria. They also tested an additional patient who had clinical signs of a drop in blood platelets after vaccination. Nearly all the patients—22 of 23—tested positive for unusual antibodies to platelet factor 4, a signaling protein that helps the body coordinate blood clotting.

The presence of the antibodies suggests that the vaccines are somehow triggering an autoimmune attack that causes large clots to form that then diminish the supply of platelets in the blood.

The study and an editorial on the cases are published in the New England Journal of Medicine.

This is at least the third study detailing the presence of these antibodies in patients with blood clots and low platelets after vaccination, and doctors say the emerging evidence suggests that doctors should remain vigilant for this new syndrome in anyone who experiences symptoms of blood clots anywhere in the body, not just the brain.

If this isn't a gaslighting clusterfuck, I don't know what is.

Hostage crisis and reprising chaos

It's April 2021, the rule of the world at this point is if you're not vaccinated your liberty to travel will be stripped. Is this a violation of human rights?

In both journalism and business school you're taught one powerful lesson. The right questions are more important than the right answers.

When it comes to gathering insights, all too often people go in knowing what they want the answer to be, rather than what the answer is.

In journalism leading questions are done intentionally like lawyers in a courtroom. In business marketing insights are important for product innovation. In the age of design thinking and preaching about agile, it seems shocking and disappointing that governments are still practising ancient ways of assuming they know best when the whole world knows that assumption is the mother of all fuckups.

People are not resistant to change. People are resistant to not knowing what and how to change. Perhaps one way to allay public fear and scrutiny is if government officials and global leaders asked the right questions:

1. Can a government compel citizens to get inoculated? Should it?
2. Should we prioritize people most likely to die from the disease (say the elderly) or those most likely to transmit it widely (say college students)?
3. Who should get the vaccine last?
4. Should healthcare workers get the first doses?
5. Should vaccines be shared with the international community?
6. Is it justifiable to deny people travel if they refuse to get vaccinated?

7. Is prioritizing the COVID-19 patients most likely to survive just?

So much could be pacified if leaders asked the right questions so the media would feed people with answers that are more communicative than information.

What's damning about this whole situation is that seventy-four years ago we had a lesson learnt called the Nuremberg Code.

The Nuremberg Code is a ten-point statement issued by the Nuremberg Military Tribunal in 1947 meant to prevent future abuse of human subjects. It states that, above all, participation in research must be voluntary. The Nazis were infamous for conducting various harmful and torturous experiments on Jewish prisoners at concentration camps. The insidious curiosity of the German doctors partly contributed to the holocaust death toll.

To this day, it remains a question as to whether all who knew of the illicit research, from German citizens to Allied forces, should be considered (or even trialled for) complicit to the crime against humanity. The Nuremberg Code aimed to protect human subjects from enduring the kind of cruelty and exploitation the prisoners endured at concentration camps. Voluntary consent is essential. The results of any experiment must be for the greater good of society. The latter however, is often manipulated as the catch-22. Identifiably people are feeling cornered to take the COVID vaccine. Unfortunately, many aren't aware of the Nuremberg Code.

The Wannsee Protocol

On 20 January 1942, fifteen high-ranking Nazi Party and German government officials gathered at a villa in the Berlin suburb of Wannsee to discuss and coordinate the implementation of what they called the 'Final Solution of the Jewish Question.' They were leaders of various Nazi ministries and organizations. The agenda was simple and focused to solve a problem: how to best eradicate eleven million Jews, some of them not living on German-controlled territory?

And like the COVID-19 vaccine rollout, the Wannsee conference had its goal but the coordination was the driver.

The 'final solution' was the codename for the systematic, deliberate, physical annihilation of the European Jews. Adolf Hitler authorized this Europe-wide scheme for mass murder. Reinhard Heydrich convened the Wannsee Conference and became legendary for this assembly. The meeting was attended by several government ministries, including state secretaries from the Foreign Office, the Justice, Interior, and State Ministries, and representatives from the SS. Of the fifteen who attended, eight held academic doctorates.

Under Heydrich's chairing, the men at the table did not deliberate whether such a plan should be undertaken, but instead discussed the implementation of a policy decision that had already been made at the highest level of the Nazi regime. Firm and harsh actions to be taken were notified in advance. They were also careful and concise about the lexicon used to describe what was to occur. Hitler was brilliant enough to be absent from this meeting. In fact all traces of this conference were to be destroyed and many euphemisms were used to camouflage it. It remains one of the world's unique examples of organizational psychology and leadership practiced with such profound global impact on the modern world.

With the support from government ministries and other interested agencies Heydrich proposed transporting Jews from every corner of Europe to concentration camps in Poland and working them to death. The leaders asked questions: What about the strong ones who took longer to die? What about the millions of Jews who were already in Poland? How do they speed the deaths of women, men, children, old, abled and disabled? How best can they physically annihilate en masse?

Although the word 'extermination' was never uttered during the meeting, the implication was clear; anyone who survived the wretched conditions of a work camp would be 'treated accordingly.'

Marvelling is the fact that the members of the conference discussed this extermination exercise with a high level of panache. It was discussed as a new policy that bypasses all recognized forms of human right violation, ethics and cruelty at the time. It was business as usual. A problem that required a solution. A means to an end.

The Wannsee Conference lasted only ninety minutes. All evidence, every piece of stationery destroyed.

The rest became history.

Lebensunwertes Leben

'An unwritten and never to be written page of glory.'
SS Heinrich Himmler,
Hitler's chief executioner

It took ninety minutes to change the course of the world.

Known as the Jewish Holocaust, the Nazis carved the audacity that there were powers that be beyond God that could designate human beings. According to their decree there were powers to determine whose lives were unimportant, or those who should be killed outright. The Germans called it *Lebensunwertes Leben*, or 'life unworthy of life'.

13.6 million soldiers believed it.

Despite well-known info on the executions, quantifying the killings remain only mere estimates up to this day. Detailed records of the killings are almost nonexistent because of the Nazis' tight secrecy around all its executions from gas, bullets to medical experiments. While Auschwitz had a reasonable number of survivors to reconstruct the history, very few survived the camps namely the three main death camps: Belzec, Sobibor and Treblinka under Operation Reinhard.

Yitzhak Arad accounts from Belzec, Sobibor, Treblinka The Operation Reinhard Death Camps:

> To accomplish the stupendous task that the Führer had set for them, they organized their camps on the model of factories; in theirs the principal product was death. Railway convoys delivered hundreds of dazed Jews, who were driven through various stations where they left behind their baggage, valuables, clothes, and finally even their hair. Deceived about the camps' purpose sometimes until the

very end (Belzec and Treblinka had camp orchestras to confuse the victims, drown out their cries and distract their murderers), they were killed in bunkers constructed to look like showers. Treblinka, the most efficient camp, could annihilate between 12,000 and 14,000 people daily, according to its commandant, Franz Stangl. Much of the ghastly work, including the disposal of the corpses, was done by Jews, who were forced into this macabre role before being killed themselves.

If it wasn't bullets, gas and intolerable cruelty, the Nazis also used the method of applied destitute. Dachau opened in 1933. It was the first German concentration camp. An estimate of 200,000 people were detained between 1933 and 1945. Known reports declare 31,591 deaths from disease, malnutrition and suicide. Alan Taylor writes in 'World War 2: the Holocaust' in The *Atlantic*: 'Unlike Auschwitz, Dachau was not explicitly an extermination camp, but conditions were so horrific that hundreds died every week.'

So horrific was the genocide that The Nuremberg trials (a series of thirteen trials carried out in Nuremberg, Germany, between 1945 and 1949 to bring Nazi war criminals, most of Hitler's head officials, to justice) led to a reassessment of international criminal law. According to the executive summary of the Nuremberg trials from Robert H. Jackson Centre:

The Nuremberg trials established that all of humanity would be guarded by an international legal shield and that even a Head of State would be held criminally responsible and punished for aggression and Crimes Against Humanity. The right of humanitarian intervention to put a stop to Crimes Against Humanity – even by a sovereign against his own citizens – gradually emerged from the Nuremberg principles affirmed by the United Nations.

But the executive summary reads a sad note:

The World Wars lead the world community to pledge that 'never again' would anything similar occur. But the shocking acts of the Nazis were not isolated incidents, which we have since consigned to history. Hundreds of thousands and in some cases millions of people have been murdered in, among others, Russia, Cambodia, Vietnam, Sierra Leone, Chile, the Philippines, the Congo, Bangladesh, Uganda, Iraq, Indonesia, East Timor, El Salvador, Burundi, Argentina, Somalia, Chad, Yugoslavia and Rwanda in the second half of the past century.(2) But what is possibly even sadder is that we, meaning the world community, have witnessed these massacres passively and stood idle and inactive. The result is that in almost every case in history, the dictator/president/head of state/military/leader responsible for carrying out these atrocities—despite being in Nuremberg—has escaped punishment, justice and even censure.

This raises the question of our value system.

The Larva comes before the Butterfly

To date, none of the COVID-19 vaccines 'made compulsory' by governments have reached full term of standard operating procedure.

According to medical literature, the overall development of a vaccine consists generally of a discovery phase, a pre-clinical phase, the clinical development phase (phases I to III) and the post licensure phase (phase IV), and it takes on average about 10-15 years. Vaccines are built on time-proven techniques. The process involves longitudinal studies, a global collaboration of experts and antigen updates (like in the case of the seasonal flu vaccines).

The COVID-19 vaccines are the exception to the rule. WHO issues all current COVID-19 vaccines under emergency use listing (EUL) validation in the pursuit for equitable global access.

In the words of WHO:

> The emergency use listing (EUL) procedure assesses the suitability of novel health products during public health emergencies. The objective is to make medicines, vaccines and diagnostics available as rapidly as possible to address the emergency while adhering to stringent criteria of safety, efficacy and quality. The assessment weighs the threat posed by the emergency as well as the benefit that would accrue from the use of the product against any potential risks.
>
> The EUL pathway involves a rigorous assessment of late phase II and phase III clinical trial data as well as substantial additional data on safety, efficacy, quality and a risk management plan. These data are reviewed by independent experts and WHO teams who consider the current body of evidence on the vaccine

under consideration, the plans for monitoring its use, and plans for further studies.

Experts from individual national authorities are invited to participate in the EUL review. Once a vaccine has been listed for WHO emergency use, WHO engages its regional regulatory networks and partners to inform national health authorities on the vaccine and its anticipated benefits based on data from clinical studies to date.

In addition to the global, regional, and country regulatory procedures for emergency use, each country undertakes a policy process to decide whether and in whom to use the vaccine, with prioritization specified for the earliest use. Countries also undertake a vaccine readiness assessment which informs the vaccine deployment and introduction plan for the implementation of the vaccine under the EUL.

As part of the EUL process, the company producing the vaccine must commit to continue to generate data to enable full licensure and WHO prequalification of the vaccine. The WHO prequalification process will assess additional clinical data generated from vaccine trials and deployment on a rolling basis to ensure the vaccine meets the necessary standards of quality, safety and efficacy for broader availability.

It is therefore with no contest that people are reluctant to be COVID vaccinated, and why should they?

With reference to the Wannsee Conference and its careful lexicography, we should remind ourselves of the goal and coordination of this COVID vaccine rollout, as spoken by a distinguished member of the powers that be, Dr Mariângela Simão, WHO Assistant-Director General for Access to Medicines and Health Products in a press release:

The World Health Organization (WHO) Emergency Use Listing (EUL) opens the door for countries to expedite their own regulatory approval processes to import and administer the vaccine. It also enables UNICEF and the Pan-American Health Organization to procure the vaccine for distribution to countries in need.

This is a very positive step towards ensuring global access to COVID-19 vaccines. But I want to emphasize the need for an even greater global effort to achieve enough vaccine supply to meet the needs of priority populations everywhere,

WHO and our partners are working night and day to evaluate other vaccines that have reached safety and efficacy standards. We encourage even more developers to come forward for review and assessment. It's vitally important that we secure the critical supply needed to serve all countries around the world and stem the pandemic.

With clear messaging of its uncertainty other than high hopes, time and luck, the vaccine rollout puts us somewhere between phase III and phase IV of the vaccine standard operating procedure. We are the rats in an open lab subject to observation in a 10-15 years ongoing clinical study. Is that the worth of my life to WHO and my government?

Taken from the US Department of Health website:

A vaccine typically contains a part of a germ (bacteria or virus) that is called an antigen. The antigen has already been killed or disabled before it's used to make the vaccine, so it can't make you sick. Antigens are substances, often a protein, that stimulate the body to produce an immune response to protect itself against attacks from future actual disease exposure. In addition, vaccines contain other ingredients that make them safer and more effective, including preservatives, adjuvants, additives and residuals of the vaccine production process. Because specific ingredients are necessary to make a vaccine, even though they are eventually removed, trace amounts can still remain. These residuals can include small amounts of antibiotics and egg or yeast protein.

So shall we discuss the blood clots?

If I refuse to be vaccinated it is not because I see COVID as a fallacy. It's because I value my life too much for blind obedience. The Führer is dead.

Flying Fxxks

I spend most of my mornings during lockdown drinking coffee on my balcony flipping through the pages of the *Edge*, Malaysia's leading business newspaper. With every lockdown someone out there is stuck between a rock and a hard place; to close or not to close his company. Those with micro-businesses depending on a daily income, such as construction workers and food sellers, they risk becoming infected or going hungry. And there were so many. Small and medium enterprises (SMEs) make up 99 per cent of the 920,624 business establishments in Malaysia, and since March 2020, have struggled the hardest to survive. These SMEs are classified into three categories: micro, small, and medium, defined by industry, sales turnover, and the number of employees. Micro-enterprises make up 76.5 per cent of Malaysian SMEs. In contrast, medium-sized enterprises comprise only 2.3 per cent of SMEs. Moratoriums and financial aid can only stretch so far. In 2021, entering our third lockdown, I was reading more incidents of business owners below forty turning to suicide.

When the pandemic hit in the first quarter of 2020 the government's blanket advice to companies was 'to pivot, embrace the new norm, and work from home'. Unfortunately, there were gaps in the advice. Pivot meant you needed to transfer businesses online and to adopt digitization. This added cost for business owners to upgrade infrastructure and to upskill employees. As a result, SMEs perform relatively poorly in digitization. There's also a digital divide among businesses in Malaysia, as SMEs are 'less likely than the average business establishment to access and use the internet' while 'large export-oriented firms dominate the digital economy as they adopt e-commerce at higher rates than SMEs' (World Bank Group, 2018).

I've always had a contention towards government-linked companies (GLCs) in Malaysia for their over-reliance on government subsidies. And now with COVID, there is economic disparity for survival. It irks me to read GLCs acting entitled for assistance at a time where people are forced to dig into their pension funds meant for their future in order to survive the present. High on the contention list is Malaysia's national carrier, Malaysian Airline Berhad (MAB). I feel compelled to share the MAB predicament because no other Malaysian GLC has been as consistently hit, criticized, yet protected for underperforming, overspending and burdening taxpayers' money. COVID-19 isn't the enemy of the state that brought many companies to their knees; it is weak leadership and poor governance that glorifies too much in its successful heydays. Henry Kissinger wrote, 'The task of the leader is to get his people from where they are to where they have not been.' MAB makes a demonstration of a broken system that struggles to do so. Perhaps if we analysed their pain points we can use them as cautionary tales to improve future businesses, including governments.

From financial losses stemming from the financial crisis in the late 1990s, disappearance of MH370 which remains unsolved but very much speculated, to the constant change of leadership, MAB is often my case study for analysing organizational practices in Malaysia. I've written essays covering five key areas: Leadership Effectiveness; Attitudes and Job satisfaction; Organizational Change Management; Staff Motivation and Equity and Justice at the workplace. While whipping the airline I take the opportunity to discuss leadership insights citing Herzberg, Maslow, Social cognitive, social learning and self-efficacy theories. (*Disclaimer: In the following chapter, note that though the company was known as Malaysian Airline Systems (MAS) till 1 September 2015 as part of a renationalization exercise, it will be known as MAB throughout the discussion.*)

Established in the 1930s under Malayan Airways Limited in Singapore, its maiden flight successfully took place in 1947 as the country was still under the British rule. After the separation of Singapore in 1963, with the formation of the Federation of Malaysia, followed by the Independence of Singapore Agreement in 1965, the company became part of Malaysian Airline System (MAS) and Singapore Airline respectively. The airline was not free of crisis although in comparison to other airlines, it was reputed being as among Asia's leading carriers, winning numerous awards such as The World's 5-Star Airlines by Skytrax in 2009, 2012 and 2013 and Asia's Leading Airline by World Travel Awards in 2010, 2011 and 2013 respectively.

In 1977 the company experienced its first crisis with the hijacking and crash of Flight 653 killing 100 people on board and most recently, the disappearance of MH370 and the gunning down of MH17 both, interestingly, within a span of four months in 2014. There have been many speculations involving political scandals, corruption and international dishonesty. However, as investigations remain ongoing, or rather, shelved to the side from the limelight, MAS which later changed to Malaysian Airlines Berhad (MAB) in 2015 was handed over to Khazanah Nasional in August 2014 seeing a series of organizational restructuring in a bid to recover its progressive losses in terms of finance and corporate image. The fact that Khazanah Nasional is a government's sovereign wealth fund did not reduce the scandal of political interferences that already mired the company. From owning 69.37 per cent of the company shares, Khazanah Nasional gradually claimed 100 per cent ownership, denationalized the airline, and delisted the airline from Malaysia's stock exchange.

Pea under the mattress

I describe the story of MAB as a quiet disaster but with a catastrophic heritage in organizational behaviour studies. On the forefront, the company remains steadfast behind its accolades and awards which claimed glory after the 1997 financial crisis pulling its reputation through the second financial crisis in 2008. However, the company has suffered a depressive reputation in terms of poor leadership that denies it financial mismanagement records supported by an equally poor misadministration in change management. And while the government continues to resuscitate its image, its management woes continue despite attempts at incorporating foreign Chief Operating Officers twice (Christoph Mueller and Peter Bellew in 2015 and 2016 respectively).

As if a curse has been placed on the company, the organizational structure remains brittle with unexpected announcements made periodically from its leaders shaking both consumers and citizens' confidence in supporting the national carrier. From rampant flight cancelations, hiked ticket prices, to biased customer service, MAB is a problematic entity.

In 2015 MAB had a total of 20,000 staff but would eventually terminate up to 8,000 employees by the end of 2016, a third of its workforce. I find it fascinating as to how a company so extensively and fully funded by the government can suffer such a prolonged period of malaise judgements and decisions that led to several waves of severe retrenchment, failed insights to botched change management strategies. My theory begins with its leadership followed by drastic restructuring that did not prepare its staff for cultural and change management styles, and lack of staff support after a series of fatal incidents televised across the globe provided them with no closure. All of these, I believe, do impinge on the overall effectiveness of staff loyalty, motivation and trust towards its leaders and management.

According to historian Thomas Carlyle a leader is 'one gifted with unique qualities that capture the imagination of the masses.' MAB saw its heyday under the leadership of Datuk Idris Jala in 2006. He engineered the 'Business Turnaround Plan' within the same year he was appointed using the Government-linked Company (GLC) Transformation Manual as a guide. Focusing on route rationalizing, Jala re-examined international routes that were not profitable and least popular, reducing domestic flights and saturated flight timings.

Jala's Project Alpha and Project Omega continued to focus on the company's network and revenue management. His strategy was to focus on six areas: pricing, revenue management, network scheduling, opening storefronts, low season strategy and distribution management. The plan worked and MAB exceeded its target by 184 per cent raking in over RM853 million in profit by Q4 of 2007.

The reputation of MAB skyrocketed redeeming its name as the proud national carrier it used to be and despite tickets sales being expensive, the airline was able to afford the image and reputation as a luxury airline with highly defined Business and First Class cabins that catered to primarily international travellers and VIPs with coveted perks and offerings. This, by large, was an effect of the Great Man theory leadership. Jala not only rescued an important but flagging entity, his strategic ingenuity impacted the airline by increasing its value by stock and reputation. Seeing the potential, the organization decides to leverage Jala's valiant status and upscale MAB's brand image.

Unfortunately, all good things come to an end. Idris Jala was called into politics, joining the cabinet in 2009, succeeded by Tengku Azmil Zahruddin as the new CEO. Riding on the exclusive image, Zahruddin went shopping. His strategy was the opposite of Jala, starting with the purchase of fifteen new Airbus A330 aircraft, with options for another ten expected to be delivered between 2011 and 2016. He expanded long-haul flights to eastern Asia and the Middle East. This was done with poor foresight as fuel prices escalated and low-budget carriers became the new option for travelling. Once again MAB was faced with financial and mismanagement difficulties, this time more serious as Zahruddin led the company into its worst financial trenches in 2011 of over RM2.52 billion (as reported by the BBC News in 2011). While Zahruddin failed to have the ethos of Jala, pressured by the epic losses, MAB became desperate to redeem its luxury image and lead-footed on the Great Man theory by appointing German CEO Christoph Mueller.

The disappearance of MH370 and explosion of MH17 highlighted the poor leadership skills of CEO Ahmad Jauhari Yahya. Immediate impact of MH370 poor crisis management led by Yahya created a substantial loss of RM307.04 million with ticket sales down by up to 60 per cent in both Malaysia and China (Reuters, 2014). According to House's Goal Path theory, a leader is substantiated by how he manages the following four aspects: leader effectiveness; environmental contingencies; employee contingencies; and leader behaviours. When MH370 disappeared, there were up to several hours of lull. During the press conference, Yahya was not the one to speak but his spokespersons.

In 2015 a press conference was to be held in Putrajaya led by Department of Civil Aviation Director-General Datuk Azharuddin Abdul Rahman to be aired live on RTM1 at 6 p.m. Abdul Rahman was to make a statement based on the 1,500-page report on the MH370 investigation. According to Information Department officer Jagjit Singh the press conference was cancelled due to 'unforeseen circumstances'. This angered members of the press and public with no further detail on what happened to the 239 passengers and cabin crew (fourteen nationalities) that disappeared on 8 March 2014 (*Star Online*, 2015). Meanwhile, Yahya remains deafeningly silent unless reading from a script. He spoke at the press conference on 7 March but not with the acumen of a CEO. He read off the script, kept limited eye contact with the audience and was informative about the passenger list not communicative in what had happened while avoiding the 'how' as there were a few hours of delay before authorities had been alerted the plane was off the Malaysian airspace radar. MAB staff were also frustrated as their friends' fate remained uncertain. This was worsened after the gun down MH17 yielded another mysterious and unexplained circumstance by the MAB authorities. As CEO, Yahya's reputation imploded and it was obvious that he was clueless to handling the unprecedented event.

As MAB continued to slip into the reds, Christoph Mueller was appointed on a three-year contract with the sole mission to mastermind a RM6.42 billion overhaul that included cutting 6,000 jobs and terminating unprofitable routes (as reported by the Associated Press in 2016). Clearly he was to be the villain in the MAB narrative. The Hersey Blanchard model is best applied here where the role of Mueller was not to establish relationships but to execute top level orders with immediate effect. Decisions are leader directed and there was no time or room for multi-tiered negotiation. Subordinates who had low levels of readiness to adopt the new foreign CEO and intense restructuring were welcomed to resign or were dismissed. In less than a year, Mueller resigned citing 'changing personal circumstances' (Reuters, 2014). Meanwhile, the fate, employment and staff trust remain hanging in the balance with more doubts, increased anxiety and plummeting leadership confidence due to Mueller's stark organizational cultural differences and lack of communication transparency in explaining the future of the organization.

Peter Bellew was appointed by the investment fund and new owner of MAB Khazanah as the next CEO post Mueller but with a different mission, to ensure continuity and further progress of the overall restructuring effort. By now the airline was on the brink of bankruptcy with Khazanah providing Bellew with RM6 billion to devise a plan to resuscitate MAB from total closure. Unlike German national Mueller, Bellew was also responsible in reviving staff confidence as the company faced a new problem: loss of employers. Taking advantage of MAB's frailty were other low-cost carriers that were growing in strength and luring experienced MAB staff with better salary schemes.

Observation of leadership behaviour shows that leaders are biased in the way they manage, communicate and treat subordinates. Ranks, division, race and culture do play a divisive role and in the case of MAB, the lower ranks were badly hit. The announcement of 6,000-job termination (a third of its workforce) was enough to rattle the confidence and dignity of the workers as MAB's sufferings and employees' fate were plastered across the media (MAB eventually terminated 8000). Khazanah not only announced a new twelve-plan strategy to remake MAB but also that they were filtering staff with a new assessment tool that was aligned with the sole company's (NewCo) new direction.

'All employees will get termination letters and either a letter to join the new company, or to register . . . [for] outplacement,' a company spokesperson told CNN. MAB's frail reputation is not a result of the two air disasters in 2014. Its problem rests on public confidence and poor understanding of organizational behavior especially from the top tier. There seems to be a major disconnect in the way top operating managers communicate with their subordinates and provide emotional support after the disappearance of MH370. Here, Maslow's hierarchy of needs is sorely neglected where organizational culture and ethics are concerned.

MH370 took 239 lives with no closure while MH17 was shot down by a Buk missile claiming another innocent 298 passengers. If death is not serious enough a call for counselling, the public announcement of terminating 6,000 jobs subsequently showed the company was ruthless and without compassion. While battling a collapsing public image, the company was also on a financial life support system to focus on what was most important at the time: staff motivation, equity and justice at the workplace. Almost overnight, MAB's cabin crew felt unsafe to fly with the national carrier. As airport security tightened due to speculation MH370 could have been hijacked by terrorists, cabin crew felt trepidation to go to work and to remain with a company that may terminate their services anyway. If we apply Maslow's hierarchy of needs, the staff tiers of safety, belonging and self-esteem were greatly shaken.

With the constant change of leadership that not only came for too short a period of time to make concrete and successful management changes compared to Idris Jala, members of staff felt demoralized and undervalued. Goals were inconsistent, future plans were discreet and it seemed obvious that MAB's priorities were to move on from the disaster as efficiently as possible to overlook media criticism that Malaysian air traffic controllers had neglected their duties. Gone were the self-determination and goal-setting theories that allowed them to be happy. Here Herzberg's 1959 Motivation-Hygiene Theory postulates that an employee's sense of belonging, their 'sequence of feelings' and what affects them (in this case the two global disasters) are what matters most to them than the Voluntary Separation Scheme (VSS). At least when the government issued a massive retrenchment exercise in 2016 where 37,699 workers were laid off, they set up the 1Malaysia Outplacement Centre (1MOC) under the Pembangunan Sumber Manusia Bhd (PSMB) which acted as a one-stop centre for Malaysian workers who were terminated. MAB failed to do so. Interestingly, this was also the same year GRAB Malaysia was activated allowing many of the terminated workers to be absorbed into the e-hailing service provider.

Still persistent in the shadow of denial to cover up misman-agement and ambiguous company practices, Deputy Finance Minister Datuk Ahmad Maslan had this to say about the termination of MAB staff, 'A bloated 20,000-strong workforce is one of the major reasons why MAS was not performing well and only 14,000 jobs is offered in the new MAB.' Statements such as this further plummet staff confidence with many questioning the RM6 billion budget and Khazanah's recovery plan which they assumed would have provided a safety net to their employment. Here, we revert to the Great Man Leadership theory. Instead of a leader, the MAS brand itself raised to luxury standards by Idris Jala as among South East Asia's top carriers refused to bend to the pressures and was willing to expense its workforce. 'They've grasped the nettle of over-employment,' said Timothy Ross, an Asian aviation analyst in Singapore for Credit Suisse as reported in USA Today. 'The airline's cultural status, and national pride, mean Malaysia won't let it die,' said Ross. 'If it wasn't for loss of face, the logical move is to close its doors.' Closure due to bankruptcy would mean the legacy of MAS and good leaders such as Idris Jala would have been removed from the great annals of Malaysian aviation history.

What confused both the public and MAB employees was the paradoxical information. On one hand you had company reps and the deputy finance minister claiming MAS had over-hired, had to lease their fleet and squeeze massively on their budget. Yet, they were giving 'extra' according to Ahmad and not what had been discussed in the Collective Agreement (CA) set by the management. 'In total, RM1.5 billion has been spent on compensation payments, securing job offers, training courses, and other benefits for employees who were terminated from MAS,' he describes. Those who worked for more than a decade get one and a half month's wage per year of service with extra benefits that include twelve months medical benefit or up until new employment is found for those who are not offered a job in MAB, employable skills training courses, entrepreneurship courses, and other workshops for retrenched employees.' Many felt that the amount spent on these 'extras' could have been cycled to ensure jobs remained rather than lost, especially to loyal staff whose knowledge, expertise and services carry more value. In relation to Herzberg's theory of motivation, 'stability and satisfaction through meaningful role, purpose and reward through sequential acknowledgement' is far more essential than being shown the door with a fat wallet.

Social learning theory shows that a powerful form of motivation and morale booster is for managers to show that workers are not just part of logistics. Transparency in communication, open communication and feedback would have perhaps provided alternatives to solving the crisis as a collective, not by selecting a handful of individuals to make drastic decisions.

It is also devastating for the staff to witness their cultural legacy, pride and heritage with MAS be dismantled and leased by a complete foreigner but that seems to be a popular strategy by multi-billion dollar companies in Asia. When criticized if it was 'healthy' to have non-locals to make big decisions over local entities such as MAB and Perusahaan Otomobil Nasional Sdn Bhd (PONSB), International Trade and Industry Minister Datuk Seri Mustapa Mohamed gave a reply that to me, perhaps intensifies the discrimination, citing 'global connections' and 'better understanding of global markets'. Mohamed explains, 'In business, it [to lead] has got to do with ability. We have to learn from each other on the best practices. I am sure those companies would not have appointed (foreign CEOs) if there was no value. They must have done a thorough analysis [before making the decision].' But if that is the case, how do you explain Mueller's short term exit? Or Bellew's persisting struggle to keep MAB afloat? What about Idris Jala? Or could it be the governmentality and constant political interferences that are the actual reasons why MAB continues to suffer?

What I admire about Idris Jala as CEO of MAS in 2005 is that he was unfazed by the unstable economy, he was transparent with his actions and he provided transparency with the release of the MAS Business Turnaround Plan (MAS, 2005) to state the company's goals, missions and timeline. He is, by all measure, a transformational leader. He was mentally, emotionally and physically prepared to lead the company through the storm. Here he begins the report by saying:

> The global airline industry is in a state of turmoil and it is increasingly clear that the survivors—and most certainly the winners—will have to make radical changes to adapt to the new environment. For FY 2005, Malaysia Airline System (MAS) reported a loss of over RM1.3 billion. This announcement came at the same time as some of our regional competitors reported strong profits. This result is unacceptable. A real business turnaround is an imperative for MAS. The new environment will continue to hit MAS hard. The projections for MAS for 2006 look dismal. In fact, on its current business assumptions, course and speed, MAS will likely fail, running out of cash in April 2006, and reporting a RM1.7 billion loss for 2006.

As a CEO he was honest about the company's position. But as a good leader with integrity and compassion for the workforce, he proceeded to write the following:

> The management team, and our staff, however, believes strongly in our ability to transform the business and, indeed, to go beyond expectations. MAS has done much to improve its performance over the last 5 years, and indeed last year. We have much to be proud of, and this work will form the foundation of our success. With hard work, radical changes and some tough decisions, MAS can certainly be a survivor and a winner. Since early December 2005, the management team has dedicated itself to the development of a plan that builds off the actions taken by the Board in 2005 to begin the turnaround. This turnaround plan will not only reverse the loss and return MAS to profitability, but also transform the company into a strong and vibrant institution—one that is capable of withstanding external shocks and aggressively tackling new opportunities.

He acknowledged the problem as a collective, and with sophisticated inclusivity he not only assured the future will be positive as a collective, but also with a strong belief that they will make it through as a collective. This, I believe, is a sterling example of citizenship behaviour and is it any wonder that with the Turnaround Plan, MAS successfully surpassed profits by 184 per cent under Jala's leadership? Better still, he was local, he was a good strategist and he understood the culture and ethics of getting his workforce to assist with the plan as a collective. He knew it was not a job for one person or a few, but as a whole team.

But the most commendable aspect of his plan was the description of how each layer of the workforce is valued as themed as The MAS Way as seen in Exhibit A.

Exhibit A: The MAS Way Framework

Number 4 of Exhibit A is what brought the workforce together without any mention of threat of termination, pessimism or doubt.

The MAS Way provides the framework for our Business Turnaround Plan:

1. **Flying to win customers**—we will reconfigure our network and our product portfolio to ensure that we have the tools and capabilities to be a top-tier player in each of the markets we serve, or we will leave.

2. **Mastering operational excellence**—we will build a unique operating capability unmatched by our peers. This capability will be reflected not only in improved operational reliability, but also in higher productivity and greater precision in everything that we do.

3. **Financing and aligning the business on P&L**—we will relentlessly increase profits with the support of a world-class Finance function that ensures true financial accountability, transparency and performance orientation in our business.

4. **Unleashing talents and capabilities**—we are committed to our people. We strongly believe that the MAS employees and managers have both the passion and talent to achieve whatever goals we set for ourselves. We will work together with our employees to ensure that they have a working environment in which their talents can thrive.

5. **Winning coalitions**—we know that we cannot achieve our goals alone. MAS needs the resolute support of the Government, its employees, managers, customers, suppliers, agents and investors. It is only with the support of these stakeholders that MAS can have the mandate it needs to make the changes that will ensure our long-term success.

The Turnaround Plan was powerful as Jala, acting as CEO, used it to remind and reinforce the cultural values and climate of MAS as a successful entity capable of overcoming obstacles. He highlights words such as 'talent' and 'capabilities' phrasing them as 'unleashing' meaning there is capability and potential for more should the task at hand be demanding and challenging. By doing so, Jala created a high-performing workforce driven by admiration for his leadership skills, and vision to succeed and turnaround the nation's beloved entity that represented an allegorical success story of the whole country.

In Jala's own words in an interview with *The Quarterly:*

Once the government agreed on what needed to be done, we made our business turnaround plan available publicly. At Shell, I never needed to do that. But Malaysia Airlines is a government-linked company and the national flagship. Publishing helped us build a winning coalition not only with the government but also with other stakeholders, like the unions, the staff, and the public. Being upfront about the P&L and making it all transparent were very important to bringing the coalition together.

Idris Jala has the acumen of a good transformational leader and this was reflected with the Transformational Report that bears his signature as a symbol of accountability. The report also bears the four distinctive characteristics of a transformational leader: inspirational, intellectual, influential and considerate. Transformational leadership can be present in any division, group, department and organization as a whole. They are brave, risk-takers and with charismatic appeal. It is to no surprise that Idris Jala was voted one of the top ten most influential policy makers in the world by Bloomberg in 2014 (as reported in Bloomberg Business in 2015). He is currently the Founder and Executive Chairman of The Global Transformation Forum (GTF), the world's singular platform for influential, global leaders to engage and share experiences and best practices on how to drive transformation. Jala was awarded the CAPA Airline Turnaround of the Year (2006) for his phenomenal turnaround feat for MAS.

Exhibit B: Characteristics of Transformational Leadership

Not all leaders are born as transformative leaders just as departments don't often possess leaders with the perfect acumen to lead. However, what can be suggested from the case study is that leaders need to be transformative by training. Jala himself had no prior background in aviation. But he had a history of turning around companies at the brink of despair while he was with Shell for twenty-three years.

All companies are not void of crisis management but the MAB case study can be exemplary of companies' best and worst practices. What disappoints me is how MAB failed to emulate what Jala has prescribed during his tenure as CEO. Instead of wiping the slate clean and placing

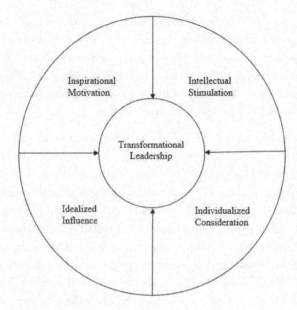

too much trust on foreign leaders they ought to have moved forward with knowledge of understanding contemporary organizational design, culture and behaviour rather than revert to traditional structures that are embedded in colonialism and imperialism narratives i.e. Europeans make better leaders.

After more than a year living with COVID-19 and watching governments at work, many old fashion ways of thinking need to be questioned. It's not just about replacing senior thought-leaders with younger whizz kids more versed with digitization, it's leadership skills. Too young and they may crumble under pressure due to insufficient experience; too seasoned and they make stubborn learners. To a certain extent I do believe Niccolò Machiavelli had it right about leadership when he wrote *The Prince* in 1513.

Machiavelli launched a thousand ships on leadership studies that even the Italian mafia refers to *The Prince* as a bible that underpins their Law of Omertà (code of silence). This may be controversial as in business and management schools, his theories are often perceived as deceitful, cunning, immoral, self-serving, dishonest or 'Machiavellian'. But seeing the world for what it is today, and at the handling of the COVID crisis, I beg to disagree. In fact, these adjectives are used within the same context of modern governing we have come to condone. Machiavelli noted five aspects of a good leader (all of which I agree):

- Should be feared rather than loved 'if you cannot be both' in order to avoid a revolt.
- Should have the support of the people because it's difficult to take action without their support.
- Should hold good virtues.
- Should never turn to outside auxiliary or mercenary units, but always rely on his (or her) own arms.
- Should be intelligent.

Interestingly, a modern leader with such virtues comes to mind. His name is Vladimir Vladimirovich Putin.

COVID: A tariff love affair?

The vaccine rollout has been argued to be a pharmaceutical ploy no different to its ancient war on cancer. In short, a market is created for supply and demand. This is a dangerous accusation but it got me intrigued as stories of new entrepreneurs were mushrooming everyday as people got laid off and created side incomes. Many friends became overnight bakers, cooks and a few tried to freelance vaccine purchases. The food was bad, most of us refused to be vaccinated, but we agreed being business mavericks was good for innovation. Stuck working from home, what else was there to do? Especially when corporate leaders kept using the word 'pivot' as part of the 'new norm'.

Long before COVID-19, the word pivot was a popularly used key term in the discourse of entrepreneurship. Entrepreneurship was a 'pivot' to the corporate manufacturing and retail business models made popular in the twenty-first century as people started to seek opportunities to initiate new businesses centred on solving communal problems, seek personal development and financial gains that could also benefit their families, and for the betterment of societies.

It became known as the business model with a conscience for the triple bottom line: people, planet and profit. And while huge corporations often had their own Corporate Social Responsibility (CSR) arm, individuals within those organisations often felt the benefit of CSR programmes were still hugely benefitting the powers that be and not the societies they're intending to help. Moreover, CSR projects are often based on the objectives and policies of the corporations rather than the communities they are funding to 'serve' and thus the seed of disruption begins.

In developing countries or better known as developing economies and bottom-of-the-pyramid markets, entrepreneurship grew exponentially with the support of angel investors and venture capitalists. The model grew popular as startups that became popular were able to scale and 'pay it forward' to newer startups by providing funding and consultancy support.

Entrepreneurship boot camps became trending in 2012 onwards as developing countries such as China and India showed how creating new opportunities for entrepreneurs to pursue was surpassing traditional manufacturing business models. Entrepreneurs became sought after careers with companies such as Alibaba, eBay and Amazon changing our views towards online retail businesses (as reported in Wall Street Journal, 2016).

Global leaders slowly paid attention and another keyword became seminal: innovation. It is believed that these private starter businesses paved the way for big new ideas, high-risk inventions and created a new excitement for a more robust and maverick-type economic climate.

Mariana Mazzucato writes a book to say this is not the case. That is the popular public misperception, 'a mythical optic' she claims, caused by poor marketing communications and lack of awareness on the term entrepreneurial leadership.

An economist and a leading figure in the area of research in innovation, Marina Mazzucato wrote a best-seller *The Entrepreneurial State: Debunking Public vs. Private Myths in Innovation* in 2013 (coincidentally the zeitgeist germinating the discourse of entrepreneurship) where she ruffled feathers but also won followers by saying that it is the federal state, or public sector, or government if you will, that is doing the following:

- leading innovation
- taking high-risks for invention
- creating, deciding and dictating the path of innovation that engines market forces.

Mazzucato states that Adam Smith's metaphorical invisible hand shaping market forces is none other than the public state, which is often described as backward, mired with bureaucratic red tape, designed to only fix problems that afflict societies at large (such as education, public health and welfare) at snail 's pace. She adds, the state is also blamed for over-regulated policies that stifle innovation. Mazzucato also outlines case studies from different sectors to show the pattern of government funding in high-level, high-stakes innovation that paves way for the private sector to glorify its success.

These areas include:

- Biotech
- Pharmaceuticals
- Green technology

Her claim is that thanks to the willingness of the federal state to take the risks and investments companies in these sectors have helped to improve not only the quality of lives, but to also provide new markets and competition that can help further engine innovation in medicine, balance its supply and demand, and push for more radical technology no private company would otherwise attempt. It also helped make these companies richer while the state remains in the shadows. But in the bigger scheme of things, thanks to the federal state for creating launchpads, many private businesses are able to thrive reaping the low hanging fruits of these innovations. And this is necessary to sustain the market that has been created.

The only problem, she says, for such high risks the state has taken, a few areas have been under-looked: financial reward and fair publicity. Taxation has been one way but there need to be more imaginative incentives for returns in perhaps forms of equity or scheme for profit sharing.

Despite this, it does not omit the fact that state-funded innovation has enabled public welfare to be improved in ways we can only imagine. The state, she says, created the groundwork necessary for the revolution of the future that is driving economies such as nanotech. And that speaks volumes on how the risks are remarkably socialised but the rewards privatised.

But how and why is there this lack of economic equilibrium? How can the state be brilliant at shaping market forces but be lacking strategy for reaping rewards? Myopic vision. This became evident in the handling of the COVID-19 crisis.

Ed Yong in his article *The COVID-19 Manhattan Project* for The *Atlantic* (who later won the Pulitzer Prize in June 2021 for his investigation) writes, 'The COVID-19 pandemic is a singular disaster, and it is reasonable for society—and scientists—to prioritize it. But the pivot was driven by opportunism as much as altruism.'

Yong describes how governments, philanthropies, and universities channelled huge sums towards COVID-19 research. The Bill & Melinda Gates Foundation apportioned $350 million for COVID work. 'Whenever there's a big pot of money, there's a feeding frenzy'.

Madhukar Pai, a fellow researcher, works on tuberculosis which causes 1.5 million deaths a year, comparable to COVID-19's toll in 2020. Yet tuberculosis research has been mostly paused. 'None of my colleagues pivoted when Ebola or Zika struck, but half of us are now working on COVID-19. Like a black hole, it has sucked us all in.'

'Science is a zero-sum game, and when one topic monopolizes attention and money, others lose out,' describes Yong. Many lines slowed to a crawl during the repeated and extended lockdowns in 2020. Many ramifications are kept away from the media. Long-term studies that monitored animals such as migration of birds or the changing of climate will forever have holes in their data because field research had to be cancelled. 'Conservationists who worked to protect monkeys and apes kept their distance for fear of passing COVID-19 to already endangered species. With experts and research volunteers stuck at home, non-COVID clinical trials were interrupted or stopped. Even research on other infectious diseases was back-burned.' For all its benefits, Yong forewarns, the single-minded focus on COVID-19 will also leave many negative legacies.

In her more recent writings (circa 2014), Mazzucato proposes a need for change: the public state ought to share the risks and rewards. Here she highlights three new key aspects: *value creation, value extraction* and *value destruction*. She also suggests green technology as the next best revolutionary way to shape a new market framework that can pivot the entire economy (as opposed to a market failure framework). Turns out it was pharmaceuticals with COVID-19.

Mazzucato has her critics. Many have argued that Mazzucato's thesis contradicts itself on her stance on industrial policy, is selective of her examples of government-funded successes, and focuses only on the capitalists' agenda that may not necessarily be for the benefit of the public but for the US military. Ideologically at its best, she lacks a convincing body of evidence to show the governance of these innovative projects that have been highly funded.

Firstly, her take on market failure is flippant. On one hand she claims that market failure is due to government policy, yet, it is also government policy that helps to create a sandbox for innovation for example in the area of orphan drugs regulation and nano technologies.

Secondly, her claim that the government inventing the internet has also been contentious. The US government has been instrumental in radical technology post World War II. In fact the US government took in several renowned scientists from Hitler's Third Reich to tap into advanced German intel experimented on Holocaust victims at concentration camps. Mazzucato lacks support for how projects are selected, expertise monitored and innovation decided for both common and market goods.

Mazzucato's belief is that it is based on the benefit of the people that so much advancement has been dedicated by the US military that led to the technological infrastructure we have for the smartphone. Critics contend however, how much of this is actually military-motivated rather than public-intended?

Popular examples provided include the iPhone which Mazzucato explains, 'though manufactured in parts by many private companies, is funded by the state to enable the technology to grow and create the smartphone market we know today.' She deconstructs the iPhone part-by-part as state-supported as follows:

The Internet - DARPA: The Defense Advanced Research Projects Agency, an agency of the United States Department of Defense responsible for the development of emerging technologies for use by the military.

GPS - The US Department of Defense and the US NAVY

SIRI - DARPA - The Defense Advanced Research Projects Agency, an agency of the United States Department of Defense responsible for the development of emerging technologies for use by the military.

Touchscreen display - Central Intelligence Agency, National Science Foundation under the US government with collaboration with the private-public owned University of Delaware.

More importantly, in connection to this, how is the distribution of grants given? How is objectivity and governance practiced that allow fair game in the playing field? How is the application of public choice theory discussed and approved?

To ardent critics, a lot of what Mazzucato is saying boils down to this: If the invention succeeds, it is thanks to the federal government. So what about the ones that failed? Do we factor that into the funding equation that had been used? As much as she amplifies the support given to the government for taking bold steps for innovation into the future, she appears naive by seeing the narrative from one positive angle and its good intention, but not as a whole. One example is the result of decentralization of industrial policy of the entrepreneurial-based SIBR programme. SIBR refers to the Small Business Innovation Research Programme acting as a central sector to risk-taking and radical growth intended to provide 'more than $2 billion per year in direct support to high-tech firms'.

Seen by critics as a taxpayer-funded venture capital, government agencies with an R&D budget over $100 million (including the military) were 'required' to spend 2.8 per cent of their budget to promote innovation by small and medium-sized businesses. This can be viewed in two ways: as a form of 'corporate hostage' and 'orchestrated tax relief scheme'. In many giant corporations over the last ten years, this can also be described as a form of CSR.

Reading *The Entrepreneurial State* and its critiques, I couldn't help but think of the following analogy; that seemingly harmless but hardworking, relevant essential worker janitor every one dismisses or silently walks by the hallway is actually Tony Stark who, when everyone is asleep cradling their Nokia 3310 teething with 3G-4G access issues is actually working on the Samsung Galaxy S Ultra with 5G technology.

Critics have argued against Mazzucato's state-infatuated claims that the federal government is the caped crusader of innovation that does not get the media credit it deserves. It is not her fault. For one, the term entrepreneur itself is problematic.

The term is problematic as not many are fully engaged with the difference of meaning, role and context between a high-investment business and a high-investment social innovation, and how the state can be represented as entrepreneurial. Why not? The only difference, if not advantage, with the public-state as opposed to private, is it has heavy backing in industrial policy, access to sufficient funding, and the necessary federal backing to see projects through while most business plans get stalled at phase one pending approval.

In this sense Mazzucato has several valid points.

One is credited to the expansion of research, and Mazzucato is a prolific researcher.

Scholars have expanded the contextual domain of entrepreneurship beyond new ventures. The term 'entrepreneurial contexts' also covers corporations acting 'entrepreneurially'. The widening of this scope legitimises the federal government to be considered as agents of entrepreneurs in

- developing new products and services
- bringing them to the market
- creating the literature and triggering competition for the market

Some have argued that companies that adopt entrepreneurial leadership tend to protect innovation that might even threaten and question industry's dominant logic, and link entrepreneurship with their strategic management.

Based on Mazzucato's belief, here the state is not. Instead, the state plays a distinctive entrepreneurial role that is key for social innovation.

- Public de-risking. Reducing the risk for big new ideas.
- Taking on the risks of high-investment innovation. Having the means and influence to pool high level funding to support two types of innovation: incremental (slow growth) and revolutionary (radical).
- Value creation. Bringing new inventions as seeds to the market and trigger proliferation.

Here, Mazzucato's work is profound by her belief that government intervention is 'not only propitious, but actually necessary for innovation to emerge'.

My support is also based on the fact that without the state's industrial policy support, patents and innovation will have low value without deployment and large-scale advocacy. The following areas have been instrumentally pushed by the government as a lead player that it has been referred to as the 'knowledge economy' for reasons of technological change, knowledge production and diffusion:

- Development of aviation
- Nuclear energy
- Computers
- The internet
- Bio and nanotechnology
- Green technology

And for this, only the federal government has power to enforce. Most private companies are risk-averse, not keen to invest in basic research, opting instead for applied research hence, the government must intervene.

Therefore in the case of COVID and vaccines, was COVID an invention to pave way for a new market for COVID vaccines? Was the virus a disruptor to force businesses to pivot into the new blue ocean? If pharma were to create a vaccine designed for a pandemic, it would require a global vaccination programme to test its efficacy. Food for thought.

I cite this case under information asymmetry. Also known as 'information failure,' information asymmetry occurs when one party to an economic transaction possesses greater material knowledge than the other party. Our market is not a free economy. With the government intervening in central planning in areas of vital importance to the nation's growth from defence, telecommunications, transportation and public health safety, information asymmetry is a necessary evil in business. It's highly deceptive, manipulated by organisations, and the best way to tackle the dissimulation is by being more empowered by how organisations are manipulating information against us.

The scarecrow, the lion and the tin man

'Opportunism, or self-interest seeking with guile, is often witnessed in human behaviour, and it bedevils human interactions and relationships.'
Dawson, Watson & Boudreau, 2014
Journal of Management Information Systems, January 2011

In the world of business, every decision and transaction involves information asymmetry. While in the push and pull of opportunities, agency theory espoused formal contracts as constraints on opportunists, information asymmetry theory is where decisions are amenable to formal contracts because one party has more or better information than the other.

I find this a very disputable grey area, stretched to great advantage by many giant organisations, experts and consultants, from top to lower level. While information asymmetry can predict adopted constraints, forestalling a decline in markets, and a host of many other researches in behaviour study, it begs many questions.

How much is allowed in suppressing information from a client?
Is hiding clauses from customers a form of legal manipulation?
How many constraints are considered non-bounded contracts?
How much is contractual?

In legal studies, information asymmetry can be considered acceptable with clauses where A is not bound to inform B which can lead to B's willingness to proceed with the contract. Deceptive, you ask? Voidability and misrepresentation can be argued, and clearly these are reasoning that make this theory controversial.

I find myself, among everyone else, stuck in this grey area between the devil and the deep blue sea, where COVID is concerned. So much data feels held against us while being funnelled like a herd of cows towards vaccination whether we like it or not. All information provided is received with skepticism. The more we are forced to accept a mandate the more the public retaliates.

'Especially when it comes to life and death questions, ethicists fiercely debate the right path—not only the path itself but the correct basis for it,' writes Jordan Kisner for the *Atlantic*.

A wide spectrum of approaches and values exists within the bioethicist community, many of them traceable to various branches of isms: An ethicist may favour deontology which suggests you should judge an action based on whether it follows moral or ethical rules such as honesty or duty to others; a consequentialist, someone who worries about the impact of a decision, as opposed to its motives; a virtue ethicist, someone whose highest priority is striving to fulfil ideals such as justice and kindness; a pragmatist, he who holds that any ethic can really be judged by evaluating its practical application; a Deweyan pragmatist, someone who believes that ethical choice evolves over time, requiring constant reevaluation; and so on.

Looking at WHO's ethical stance (as with all standards of public health emergencies) the call to action is 'just try to save as many lives'. But to what measure?

Cross-selling lives

If information asymmetry is the lingua franca of the business world, and COVID vaccination is part of the business world, then how are we to survive it in order to succeed? Answer is by understanding how to play by the rules and knowledge of the game. We can take the cue from Ping An.

Ping An is China's second largest insurer and biggest non-state owned company by revenue. Known for its high investment in its innovation arm (company earmarks 1 per cent of their revenue for investments in innovation), Ping An has over 15,000 patent technology applications operated by a team of 24,000 software engineers, 800 data scientists and 180 Artificial Intelligent specialists.

Here's how they did it. They took the old-fashion process of insurance claiming, removed standing in line and time filling up forms, and replaced it with a 'Superfast Onsite Investigation' system accessible via smartphone app. Policy holders just have to snap photos of the damaged vehicle, answer a few questions, and send them to a Ping An computer, which will respond with a repair estimate in less than three minutes, and once the customer agrees, funds are transferred immediately. You don't have to wait for an inspector as Ping An trusts its customers 'because we have been doing this for years,' says Jessica Tan, Ping An's Deputy CEO of technology.

In 2018, Ping An was able to settle 7.3 million worth of claims (62 per cent of the total). Impact to this is it saves up to 750 million each year by reducing fake claims and human error. The best part is Ping An matches photos of vehicle damage against a database of twenty-five million parts used in 60,000 auto makers and models sold in China.

Costs of parts and labour are calculated based on more than 140,000 garages integrating voice, face, and image recognition tech that can detect if customers are lying when submitting their claims. But there is a lot that customers are not aware of.

Ping An's colossal success is due to its smart virtuous circle of big data cloud involving big ticket transactions affecting meaningful decisions in customers' lives: health, wealth, property. This makes Ping An a favourite among financial institutions—200 banks to be precise. The data helps cross-sell lucrative products. For example when people use Autohome to buy a car, they wind up getting insurance from Ping An. Data into health allows the Chinese government to have a predictor of an onset of chronic diseases; 54 per cent of males smoke, 9 per cent of long term smokers get lung cancer, and a host of other diseases related to obesity, lack of exercise and heart disease.

The company is now helping the government to digitize medical records, analyse health data, pay bills and spot fraud (currently the Chinese government covers 55 per cent of the country's health care costs). But the catch-22 is, decisions on loans and insurance for individuals are currently not anonymous and have no privacy rights. Unlike the West, China has little regard for data privacy. Weibo is a good example of how the government data tracks the digital footprints of its citizens' Orwellian style.

China is infamous for information asymmetry as a way to overtly express the governments' control over its citizens. This is supported by giants like Ping An who benefit from this symbiotic relationship by sharing their cloud data. In this sense, the citizens have no power over their decisions. They are at the mercy of a Machiavellian system that operates like Bentham's Panopticon theory, where people will obey prevailing rules and norms when they know they are being watched.

In Malaysia, the vaccination rollout became a clusterfuck because of high-level distrust towards the government. The distrust impacted the national vaccination programme that people were refusing to turn up or to even register for their mandated jab. As of 25 June 2021 out of a population of 32.7 million, only 6.3 million COVID-19 vaccine doses had been administered since the beginning of the vaccine rollout in March, with 1.73 million people fully vaccinated. This means merely 14 per cent of the population have at least received their first dose. This slow and disgruntled crawl had to do with the fact the government kept extending the lockdown (another two weeks, folks, and another two) to daunt and drive out citizens from their homes to get jabbed or to remain under house arrest. 'We need to reach herd immunity,' they say. But to many it was beginning to feel like a hostage situation. Pawan Mishra, author of *Coinman: An Untold Conspiracy* wrote, 'A breach in trust brings mistrust, followed by a multitude of troubles.' Indeed this became the problem.

Influenced by the western media, skeptical citizens turned to Twitter to demand options such as Ivermectin, an anti-parasitic drug mostly used in veterinary medicine to treat worm infestations. In April 2020, researchers using laboratory methods showed that Ivermectin can also inhibit the replication of SARS-CoV-2, the novel virus that causes COVID-19 illness. Problem is, as reported by the Ministry of Health, many Ivermectin studies had limitations including small sample size, non-controlled study designs or that the drug was used as add-on treatment. 'Therefore this had confounded the effect of Ivermectin, if any.' Once more the house was divided. Regulatory bodies including the US FDA and the European EMA, after evaluating these studies, have concluded that there was insufficient evidence to support the use of Ivermectin as treatment of COVID-19. The WHO also issued guidelines against the routine use of Ivermectin in the treatment of COVID-19 except in clinical trial settings. But all these were shared and circulated by citizens. The government tried to sound reluctant. They had enough problems of their own—vaccine shortage.

On 12 January, after persuasion from Prime Minister Tan Sri Muhyiddin Yassin, the Yang di-Pertuan Agong Al-Sultan Abdullah Ri'ayatuddin Al-Mustafa Billah Shah, the country's monarch issued a proclamation of Emergency throughout Malaysia that takes effect from January 11 to August 1. The Emergency Proclamation was made under Article 150(1) of the Federal Constitution to curb the spread of COVID-19. It took the nation by surprise. In his speech, the prime minister said: 'I appeal to you brothers and sisters to remain calm and give full trust and support to the government throughout the emergency period.' He also promised that he will not abuse Emergency powers to interfere with the judiciary, which is to function as usual. 'The judiciary will continue to be the beacon of justice in our country and I will never interfere in the business of the court,' he said in his speech. Within months, distrust increased, tensions flared. Citizens turned to their socmed platforms to exchange angst after a series of questionable decisions made by leading ministers. The hashtag **#kitajagakita** (as we look after each other) became emblematic to criticize the government accused of suppressing information on government spending (a sum of RM70 mil was used to create the problematic app for vaccine rollout), misappropriating taxpayers' funds and refusing to reopen its parliament. Turns out with the Declaration of Emergency, we all got punk'd.

As reported in the *Malay Mail*:

Under the Emergency declaration, Parliament and state legislative assemblies will not be meeting, until such a time as decided by the Yang di-Pertuan Agong. This means that lawmakers, both at the state and federal levels, will not be able to make new laws or change any existing law. Parliament and state assemblies are also important places where elected representatives ask the government for answers on policies, action and also data, while motions such as to measure confidence levels in the government can also be voted on there.

In suffering we rake our profit

In a 2015 documentary titled *24 and Ready to Die* produced by the *Economist*, audiences are educated on their options to die. Assisted death was originally seen as a 'treatment' for patients with terminal illness and unbearable pain certified by experts to be incurable by medical science.

As of 2014, Belgian laws not only allow patients with mental health to be given the option for assisted death, but also minors with the consent of their parents. This triggers human rights advocators to scream unjust murder as mental health is difficult to be scientifically proven by X-ray or tangible proof. Based on speculation, patients merely need the approval of three experts and a date can be set for their 'death'.

A contention raised after the documentary was aired was why was the *Economist* producing the story?

This led to a deeper investigation on how the business of euthanasia is a game of information asymmetry where the doctors are in absolute control to manipulate the mental health of a patient into thinking he is best to take the option to die (taken from the Patients Rights Council, 2014).

One must also remember that assisted death is also a form of medical treatment which includes doctor's visits, counselling sessions and ultimately the lethal injections administered to the patients. All of these are paid for by the patients as part of a pathway programme towards death. Protestors argue that the doctors using their ethos as medical experts onto the patients is dangerous. Patients who are already in vulnerable states are positioned under a form of duress to make decisions that could be reversed with a different intervention or alternative palliative care.

I feel that while in business information asymmetry is necessary to create the supply and demand scale, there should be conditions or rules to the norm. One of them is to disallow the weak and this includes the entire healthcare industry namely pharmaceuticals.

People who are suffering, who are under duress, or with little financial means are easy prey to a system that ought to focus on those who are more privileged. The same reason why it does not make sense holding people as hostage for vaccination if they are unsure, depriving them of aid that they have no choice but to pocket into their own pension funds, or that the 10 per cent wealthy be given so much tax relief just because they are seen to be contributing to the development of nations and the global economy.

In the Bronx, doctors noticed patients who are most vulnerable to COVID-19 are people of colour, the uninsured, and the Medicaid recipients. Writes Jordan Kisner in *The Committee of Life and Death*, 'In such areas hospitals drafted doctors from other specialties into critical care, turned conference rooms into intensive care units, built tents outside to test and triage patients, reused PPE when possible, and retrained staff on alternative ventilation equipment.'

The fear was not people dying in droves from COVID-19 but from lack of ventilators, dearth of PPE and overstretched medical staff, writes Kisner. It's the human errors. And with the vaccines creating unprecedented problems such as blood clots and unexplained deaths this places a bigger toll on the community as a whole. Haven't we been taxed enough financially, psychologically and now physiologically?

When death wasn't knocking on Heaven's door, it was giving out Golden Tickets. Towards the end of 2020, talks were heating up about vaccine passports. *Bloomberg* calls it 'The Golden Ticket' signifying your access to freedom beyond what are currently closed borders. Vaccine passports are certificates or digital cards testifying to the apparent low-risk of their holders. And while COVID may linger on for years, there are countries that are heavily dependent on tourism, from Thailand, Maldives to the Caribbean. And they need to reopen ASAP.

Greece was willing to welcome guests as early as May 2021, as long as they have been vaccinated. Boat rentals almost came to a close on the island. The holiday sector accounts for almost a quarter of Greece's gross domestic product before the pandemic, the highest proportion in Europe. The International Air Transport Association estimates the industry could lose $95 billion (USD) in cash in 2021, the worst on its record.

Aside from COVID passports, airlines will also need to support tech solutions to verify passengers' COVID vaccination, or at least verify testing results, such as the IATA Travel Pass app or the AOKpass from French travel security company International SOS[4].

In Israel, users of the government's 'green pass' mobile app can permit citizens to enter theatres, sporting arenas, hotels and gyms. The app will show they've had their vaccine shots or recovered from the virus. All these apps are currently undergoing limitations presenting high risk for forgery and data leakage.

These digital cards are not just about COVID-19 anymore. Engineers are hoping in the future they work as health and security passes to allow people to present proof of immunization such as yellow fever and kids' school registration against human trafficking. The issue standing is to filter the access so border agents gain entry only to the necessary verified information restricting personal data on central servers. Great as this sounds, the vaccine passports risk leaving behind the poorest and most vulnerable.

'What sounds like a practical solution to an unprecedented problem opens the door to a host of ethical and legal concerns,' describes United Kingdom's Conservative MP Steve Baker in a parliamentary debate. 'I did not think that is the society that we wished to live in.' This isn't a problem just for the politicians. Ethicists and epidemiologists are grappling with the issue centred on equity. The way the passports are prescribed it sounds like it could benefit the wealthy and more fortunate while leaving behind the minority groups and the poor. This could widen social divides even bigger than pre-pandemic days. Companies that mandate 'no jab, no job' face legal risks and can be tested in court.

---

[4] EU is working on its EU Digital Green Certificate, the International Air Transport Association's Travel Pass or CommonPass, backed by the World Economic Forum.

Perhaps the biggest concern at this point should be our main priority: access to vaccines. This applies most to the poorest and developing countries that stand furthest from holding a golden ticket. In a documentary on the ultra rich in Germany, *Germany: The discreet lives of the super rich* by *DW Documentary* (where many remain unknown and shy from the media spotlight) one successful entrepreneur said it best:

> In Germany, it matters less how one is rich. It matters more that the rich and those who are successful can help distribute the wealth to develop their communities like build schools, improve free education and health care. The goal is to reduce the social divide to avoid becoming like the United States. Wealth has no value until you put it to good use.

In Change we trust

'Effective change communication is at the heart of successful change, it acts like the blood in our bodies, but instead of supplying vital oxygen and nutrients, communication supplies information and motivation to the impacted stakeholders.'
Peter F. Gallagher

As the economy becomes brutally ravaged by COVID-19, one does not live without discussing the paradox of how companies need to thrive in the face of new adversities. Prior to COVID-19 companies were pressured to scale and face challenges such as industry 4.0 and the digital transformation it brings. The pandemic merely hastened the speed and need for change management.

Change management has many different guises. Project managers view change management as the process used to obtain approval for changes to the scope, timeline, or budget of a project. Infrastructure professionals consider change management to be the process for approving, testing, and installing a new piece of equipment, a cloud instance, or a new release of an application. From an organizational perspective, leaders look at the human side of change in organizational contexts.

Change management is inevitable with intimidating challenges such as stress, systems change, organizational restructuring, and leadership. If you are a manager, you are also a change agent. Businesses affected by the pandemic, on occasions would have been mired in the volatile interplay of motivation, power and politics, organizational change and most common to all, stress management. Many by now, would have had to endure letting go of good people, moving into a smaller office, working in no office, and the hardest task of all: leading whatever's left towards new frontiers.

> 'The competitor to be feared is one who never bothers about you at all, but goes on making his own business better all the time.'
>
> —Henry Ford

An organization that faces no struggle is one of the following two: one, a mythical entity close to non-existence; two, one that is stagnant with muted problems.

A healthy organization is robust and fraught with daily operational challenges that require action, decision-making and continuous efforts of housekeeping, pandemic or no pandemic. It sounds like a lot of work but that is clearly what it takes to manage a building of multi-tiered relationships and an efficient stakeholder management. Tom Gimble, founder and CEO of LaSalle Network, a top employment agency in Chicago, describes 'A good company gets the work done, but a great company stays proactive.' But what scares and stresses managers are the very reasons why they allow themselves to stay ahead of their competitors and improve profits. In times of corona, change has now become part of the new norm. How do we even begin?

Managers are change agents. What they say and do create ripples of effect that wave top to bottom and across departments. Organizational management is more relevant today than ever as modern and global business ethics require us to be more agile, cross-culturally perceptive and open to systems change. Rob Liano, author of *Counter-Attack* writes, 'You must embrace change before change erases you.'

> 'You don't have to be great to start, but you have to start to be great.'
>
> —Zig Ziglar

Three contexts are inevitable to every leader: motivation; power and politics; and organizational change and stress management. It is interesting to note that most motivational quotes present a binary opposition of circumstances: success versus failure; begin versus end; top versus bottom; up versus down; need versus desire. To a large extent that is how corporate organizations have come to perceive and measure motivation when it comes to work performance. What is missing is the mid-section to what constitutes the value, quality and process of the desired motivational outcome. In organizational management studies Maslow's hierarchy of needs creates the bedrock of understanding what drives us, what are our needs, and how we prioritize them (see image below):

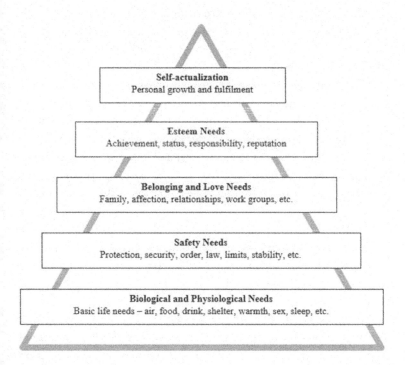

Another contention I feel that needs to be seriously considered, namely by HR management, is the fact that individual personalities, beliefs, goals and values affect the way we address motivation. Hence, we cannot see it as one framework that fits all. Other is company and department culture, gender and climate of generation.

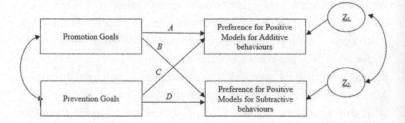

According to the Self-Determination and Goal-Setting Theory, people differ in the way they regulate their thoughts towards achieving their goals. They can be divided into two categories: promotion focus and preventive focus.

Based on the image above, people who are promotion-focused will strive for advancement and accomplishment in the pursuit of achieving their goals. They are open to opportunities and are willing to go above and beyond the call of duty to show other capabilities with the potential to upscale sooner than later. Those who are preventive-focused will aim to fulfil their duties while avoiding conditions that could pull them away from their goals. They are task-oriented due to their cautious nature, and believe in being responsible to what is given to them from their managers out of respect and obedience. One can deduce that promotion focus people are more self-driven and with high potential staff qualities to be leaders; while prevention focus staff would prefer stability and consistency in order to be efficient at their job.

Another aspect of motivation is volition. Volition is described as the strength of will needed to complete a task, 'the diligence of pursuit.' A variety of distractions and pulls of opportunities can derail a person from his job. A better offer from a competitor, personal pursuits such as to travel, a colleague who resigns from the same company are examples that can distract an employee. Kuhl in his 1987 book *Action Control: The Maintenance of Motivational States* argues that many case studies on motivation ignore the volitional processes that include these distracting factors.

'While a weak leader has a proclivity to please the critics and the leeches, a strong leader has no qualms about what the enemies say about him or his style of governance, but what intrinsic benefit does his ethical and political action bring toward the highest and common good of his people.'

—Danny Castillones Sillada

With regard to power and politics, it used to be a natural acceptance for a leader to decide over his people. History narrates to us how leaders were born into their roles and led their troops into battle, which in direct translation meant directly to their death. No one contested and no one suggested a vote for dissent. This was the rule but today we question the morality, the ethics and the humanitarian aspect of such leadership and blind obedience.

In today's corporate setting, the general dependency postulates that when you possess what others need but only you control, you gain power over them. You wear the cloak of invincibility. Wrongfully used, you end up corrupted with greed and become a dictator. Image below describes the directional influences of power tactics that are commonly found in a corporate organization.

Preferred Power Tactics by Influence Direction

Upward Influence	Downward Influence	Lateral Influence
Rational persuasion	Rational persuasion	Rational persuasion
	Inspirational appeals	Consultation
	Pressure	Ingratiation
	Consultation	Exchange
	Ingratiation	Legitimacy
	Exchange	Personal appeals
	Legitimacy	Coalitions

How a leader applies power tactics reflects on his maturity, experience and ability to strategize. Whether you're a leader in a corporate organization or an SME, one can be easily corrupted if he lacks the maturity to see the difference between influencing others and dominating others. Another indicator of immaturity is when power is given to someone too young he will not be able to lead and manage his team which includes overlooking internal training and development of individuals, growth of department, daily operations and stakeholder management.

The death knell comes in the form of decision making. I have experienced many managers who are indecisive and falter at critical moments when a firm or executive decision has to be made. The most successful leaders are the ones who do not flaunt their power through imposition but through adaptation. They are able to provide empathy and compassion where needed and when times are tough, stand by the team and are willing to take accountability of their actions, even if the outcome is not desirable.

There are strategies to decrease the potential of over-inflated power of a leader in a department, or to spread the risk of imbalanced leadership. One strategy is to apply Agile. The current buzzword for revolutionary approach to project management and product development, Agile organizations are 'self-organizing, cross-functioning teams that move away from the traditional waterfall methodology of corporate management,' and they learn to experiment and adapt by rapid iterations, in what is described as in lock-step with evolving customer needs.

Needless to say, since its presence in 2001 in the area of software development, it is now suggested for C-level executives, or anyone holding a magnitude of executive responsibility. But while Agile is designed for customer-centricity, would this approach work for a board of directors with the gamut of stakeholders? 'Directors are expected to take into account the interests of all stakeholders—shareholders, employees, customers, suppliers, etc.—in a way that serves the company itself and ensures its sustainable development. Unlike Agile product development teams, directors should not rush to appease any particular stakeholder but strive to ensure harmony.'

Agile can be successful with leaders if the strategy focuses on two key changes: one, switch from calendar-based planning process to continuous issue-based planning and; two, see the executive team as an Agile scrum. Steve Jobs and Jeff Bezos applied Agile which allowed the power shift of making decisions—while allowing space for decisions to be wrong—and led the team to spend more time on strategy, competitor actions and timely responses.

Bezos highlights a good strategy to efficient leadership management called course corrective. He describes:

> Most decisions should probably be made with somewhere around 70 percent of the information you wish you had. If you wait for 90 percent, in most cases, you're probably being slow. Plus, either way, you need to be good at quickly recognizing and correcting bad decisions. If you're good at course correcting, being wrong may be less costly than you think, whereas being slow is going to be expensive for sure.

> There are 3 groups of employees in any change journey: 'Advocates', 'Observers' and 'Rebels'. Each reacts differently to organisational change and will have different levels of resistance'
> —Peter F. Gallagher

All companies will need to change. The question is, will they act on it? Nokia remains the infamous cautionary tale in the discourse of change management. Originating from Finland, Nokia controlled 40 per cent of the mobile phones industry. They were everywhere and they were hardy. Nokia phones were described as user-friendly and the ringtones developed a personality and tonality for being omnipresent.

While the story on the street was Nokia grew over-confident and complacent, from a management standpoint that is not quite the case. Nokia committed two mistakes which many companies are currently at stake of emulating: delay in finding the 'third leg' and; too absorbed in managing growth in existing areas than finding new growth.

By the time they got around to their competitors, they lagged too far behind not due to lack of capacity building, but due to timing. Under Nokia's top management team was an internal department called Nokia Ventures Organization (NVO). The internal department was created similar to a cross-breed of research and development and learning and development. Operating like an innovation lab, NVO were actually ahead of technological advancement; they were among the pioneers to correctly identify the Internet of things (IoT). NVO also discovered a new growth area in multimedia health management. Sadly, they didn't act on the advancement. Reason being top management felt it was more worthy of their time and investment to focus on their short-term performance requirement (which ironically was very traditional in thinking) versus long-term nature of activities.

Nokia was also overly confident with their data which showed a high level of loyal customers and share positioning. However, their CEO at the time Jorma Ollila grew concerned about their loss of agility and entrepreneurialism. These two words were going to haunt them for a long time. Between 2001 and 2005 Nokia was set to rekindle their charm among mobile users. Unfortunately, what led to their decline was not what happened in the outside world among their consumers. It was internal. Nokia made a critical error by repositioning leaders and poorly reorganizing themselves into a matrix organizational structure. Vital leaders exited leading to a loss of strategic thinking.

A matrix organization structure has its pros and cons. Advantages include staffers being able to autonomously self-manage between competing bosses, and this enhances motivation and decision-making. Disadvantages include conflicting pull on resources, overlapping processes or procedures leading to turf battles and lack of accountability. A matrix organization is considered the toughest organizational form to work in and it was the last thing Nokia needed in the development of change of product development, user experience and consumer habits. The internal collapse and spiralling into their own processes cost them to be sold to Microsoft in 2013. Unfortunately, that too could not revive the once mighty giant.

By today's standards, business as usual is changing. The way companies operate has presented new indicators for stress ranging from IoT, digital transformation and operating across continents and cross departments with different time zones and work culture. Kotter presents an eight-step mechanism to ease major shifts at the workplace. Although it breaks into eight steps, it provides almost identical effect to Lewin's three-way model.

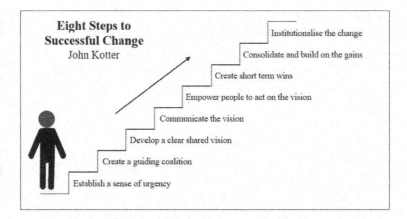

'People don't resist change; they resist being changed.'

—Frank Sonnenberg

Change management is not easy if not handled with care. Every organizational change presents anxiety and stress for the staff. Problem with being human, we are creatures of habit accustomed to thinking in a linear structure, hence, when a daily operational processing is disrupted, some people can't handle the unfamiliarity. This includes a change of leadership, procedures, merging of departments or even termination of departments.

Kurt Lewin's model for change (see model below) is broken into three parts: unfreeze; change and; refreeze. The purpose of the unfreeze stage is to allow space and time for the dismantling of old ways of doing things. Unfreezing is also critical to create awareness by the people that will be affected by the change. The employees must feel involved and accept that a better way of doing things is the better option, and that this would help to reduce levels of stress from the lack of current work problems. The management has to show the employees the logic, value and the competitive edge this necessary change brings to them. Once they are unfrozen, they can move into this new state of being. Transitioning and moving is marked by the change. People may struggle with reality and this could be stressful for some. Each stage presents a fair amount of stress and how the employees respond, react and recover from this stage is paramount to how discerning the management is towards the needs and goals of staff. The more prepared they are during the unfreezing stage the better in order to prevent them from being overwhelmed by, or resenting, the change. Communication and support are crucial at this point.

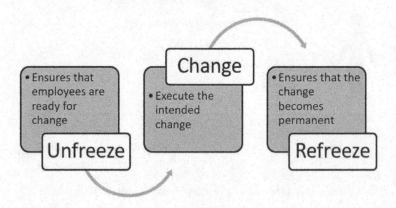

The most succinct description was given by Yves Doz, Emeritus Professor of Strategic Management at INSEAD, where he said, 'The biggest disruptive threat to a mature, successful company's future is its own success.' This can be seen in the case of Kodak, Blockbuster, and Malaysia's very own Malaysian Airlines Berhad. At the height of their success, they became risk averse and less innovative caused by a composite of what I call *The Constantinople Distraction*, poor strategic decisions due to a decline in the strategy process simply because the powers that be were looking in the wrong direction[5].

---

[5] Inspired by the infamous fall of Constantinople, which marked the end of the Byzantine Empire, the Medieval period, and effectively the end of the Roman Empire, a state which dated back to 27 BC and lasted nearly 1,500 years. Led by Mehmed II who was barely 20, Europe hoped his inexperience would lead the Ottomans astray. But his actions spoke volumes. To distract the enemies coming from the sea, Mehmed ordered the construction of a road of greased logs across Galata on the north side of the Golden Horn, and dragged his ships over the hill, directly into the Golden Horn. You read right. Ships over the hill. Mehmet was an early example of an empowering leader who was agile, innovative and with a growth mindset.

And to leaders enduring hard times such as COVID-19, it becomes imperative to see the magic and gold in muddied waters despite the current of adversities. If COVID has taught us anything about change management, it's that the industrial model does nor work anymore. Amit Ray, author of *Mindfulness Meditation for Corporate Leadership and Management* writes, 'Adaptability and change management requires strong emotional and social intelligence. It is a part of inside-out leadership.' This is true. Perhaps working nine-to-five isn't necessary. Perhaps a three-day weekend can produce happier workers. Perhaps COVID-19 is a reminder that the way we are living our lives on autopilot was the disease. Perhaps being retrenched means you're given a chance to fulfil the dream you buried. Perhaps working remotely is teaching businesses to adopt more creativity rather than flexibility. Perhaps it is time for leaders to stop instructing and to start listening. 'Fixed mindset leaders will quickly contaminate an organisation by killing growth and creativity, as well as promoting incompetence based on their likeness. This cycle will be replicated unless shareholders intervene ruthlessly,' warns Peter F. Gallagher, in *Change Management Leadership: Leadership of Change*. Indeed this could be the renaissance for leaders to unlearn and relearn.

COVID: The rich caused it

'Medicine is a social science.'
Rudolph Virchow

In 1848 a young physicist was sent by the Prussian government to investigate a typhus epidemic in Upper Silesia, Poland. He went clueless to what caused it but he soon discovered reasons for how and why it spread: broken social systems.

Virchow's report was insightful. It showed social inactions rather than actions: malnutrition, hazardous working conditions, crowded housing, poor sanitation and most wicked of all, lack of conscientiousness and repudiation for civic mindedness by civil servants and aristocrats.

Writes Suzy Kassem in *Rise Up and Salute the Sun: The Writings of Suzy Kassem:*

> To really change the world, we have to help people change the way they see things. Global betterment is a mental process, not one that requires huge sums of money or a high level of authority. Change has to be psychological. So if you want to see real change, stay persistent in educating humanity on how similar we all are than different. Don't only strive to be the change you want to see in the world, but also help all those around you see the world through commonalities of the heart so that they would want to change with you. This is how humanity will evolve to become better. This is how you can change the world. The language of the heart is mankind's main common language.

But then science got in the way.

In the pursuit of being objective, scientists in the nineteenth century felt societal factors were not definitive to explain reproduction numbers. It was soft science, an estimate at its best, especially when pitted against microbe discovery via germ theory that was making waves in the area of cholera, dysentery and syphilis.

Unfortunately, as witnessed in the case of COVID-19, data have pointed to living standards, nutrition and sanitation. We see a rapid resurgence in social medicine.

COVID-19 has been controversial not just for its virulent nature but for questioning socio-political standards.

Since March 2020 politicians and global leaders have been pacing back and forth for diplomatic answers to placate nations of unrest. Initially describing the outbreak as an equalizer, a reset, or a turning point for a new normal, eventually the truths could no longer be ignored: the disease was killing people on the margins. People who had more health problems meant they had less access to health care. Victims included those from the poor neighbourhood where responses from the health department took up to five days. They were also essential workers, migrant workers, and people living in cramped and crowded spaces that compromised both their lives and livelihood.

'These disparities aren't biological,' writes Ed Yong in *The Manhattan Project*. 'They stem from years of discrimination and segregation that left minorities in poorer neighbourhoods with low-paying jobs and less access to healthcare, the same problems raised by Virchow 170 years ago.' For the migrant workers and refugees, it was also the fear to reach access due to their illegal status or lack of identity papers. Dependent on their employers, many were left to fend for themselves when showing symptoms, more fearful of losing their jobs than risking their lives.

That's a problem on one end of the social spectrum. We have more heading towards us in the future from the middle income.

Sweden was reluctant to shut down schools to the chagrin of many other countries. But there are lessons to learn there.

'Disrupting a child's schooling at the wrong time can affect their entire career,' says Whitney Robinson of University of North Carolina. 'Think about critical periods that can affect the trajectory of your life.

Scientists should have prioritized research to figure out whether and how schools could open safely.'

But were scientists referred to before political leaders made their call? Doubtful. In fact once online teaching and learning were deemed convenient (as long as everyone stayed home the situation was under control), it became 'out of sight out of mind.' The rule of thumb was the less people we had walking around in schools the better. But then another problem was poorly examined; internet capacity of those in crowded homes, poorer neighbourhoods and those deprived of hardware and gadgetry. Indeed, intellectual brainstorming was insubstantial and again, if it's not a problem for the rich and afforded, the situation is under control. Out of sight, out of mind.

A mistake by many governments was to overprioritize COVID-19.

'To study COVID-19 is not only to study the disease itself as a biological entity,' says Alondra Nelson, the president of the Social Science Research Council based in the United States. 'What looks like a single problem is actually all things, all at once. So what we're actually studying is literally everything in society, at every scale, from supply chains to individual relationships.'

Known as social epidemiology, the mistake we're making is looking at the scabs on the surface of the skin ignoring the deeper layers that contribute to the pain and recovery. And this attitude needs to change, says Yong 'because vaccines will not immediately end the pandemic.' Even after we achieve herd immunity, the virus will still circulate. 'Outbreaks may be sporadic and short lived. The world of vaccine development will not be the same again.' But we cannot negate the slew of social and psychological ramifications it leaves behind.

We also cannot afford to drop everything, suspend the daily runnings of society allowing its economy to collapse, in the pursuit of solving one problem. COVID-19 should be a lesson of distributing risks, crisis management and shared leadership.

Aside from the myopic vision and approach, the rush and haste were also damaging.

'Flawed research made the pandemic more confusing, influencing misguided policies,' explains Yong. From fall 2019 to date, PubMed lists over 74,000 COVID-related scientific papers, more than twice for polio, measles, cholera and dengue. By September 2020, *New England Journal of Medicine* received 30,000 submissions centreed on COVID-19. However, quantity does not guarantee quality let alone accuracy and this has created a ripple effect to the information trickled to the public. Adds Yong, 'Overconfident poseurs published misleading work on topics in which they had no expertise. At its worst, it is a self-interest pursuit of greater prestige at the cost of truth and rigor.'

And all this streams to corrupt and incompetent politicians and ministers who further distill the data to their advantage.

Indeed COVID-19 itself has been victimised by the powers that be. Perhaps the situation could have been meted out with less drama and severity. Perhaps more lives could have been saved than lost.

Rudolf Virchow was horrified by his discovery that he advocated for social reforms. He tried, at least. And now it is our turn to push for social reforms within our own capacity to fix our broken systems. We need to fight against warped incentives, social inequality and in the event of another pandemic, a biomedical bias. Looking at our bank accounts, we can no longer afford it.

' . . . things are never as complicated as they seem. It is only our arrogance that prompts us to find unnecessarily complicated answers to simple problems.'
—Muhammad Yunus, *Banker to the Poor: Micro-Lending and the Battle Against World Poverty*

End Note

Normally, when you challenge the conventional wisdom—that the current economic and political system is the only possible one—the first reaction you are likely to get is a demand for a detailed architectural blueprint of how an alternative system would work, down to the nature of its financial instruments, energy supplies, and policies of sewer maintenance. Next, you are likely to be asked for a detailed program of how this system will be brought into existence. Historically, this is ridiculous. When has social change ever happened according to someone's blueprint? It's not as if a small circle of visionaries in Renaissance Florence conceived of something they called 'capitalism,' figured out the details of how the stock exchange and factories would someday work, and then put in place a program to bring their visions into reality. In fact, the idea is so absurd we might well ask ourselves how it ever occurred to us to imagine this is how change happens to begin.
—David Graebe, American anthropologist and anarchist activist

Needless to say, we are currently living in very interesting times. Times which cannot be undone or unwritten, blocked or unpost, only lived and to be reflected upon.

I wrote this with the introduction of this manuscript in mind. Then I felt it did more poetic justice as a conclusion. As a reminder to embrace the unknown and the uncertain, as ways to harness our emotional intelligence. It is perhaps the most critical type of intelligence we need to hone and to promote in today's climate.

I truly believe COVID-19 is a blessing more than a bane. Writing this I am still under lockdown, a situation I thought I would have escaped by now. After fifteen months it has brought a sense of fulfilment, a jolt out of the mundane in between the low grade depression. In the wise words of Viktor Frankl, 'The greatest human achievement is not success, but facing an unchangeable fate with great courage.'

On days I wake up feeling the weight of the world on my shoulder, I remind myself I am not alone in this. There are more stories out there to be researched, to look into and to reflect upon. My higher voice pacifies I've entered day 456. Anne Frank survived 761 in a tight annex. Outside from my balcony I visualize the blue yonder. I can smell the salty coast of Portofino. A bigger world awaits. A better version of me stands taller today, my back straight, shoulders relaxed, and chin up. 'The neocortex allows for the subtlety and complexity of emotional life, such as the ability to have feelings about our feelings.' writes Daniel Goleman. 'It's not the highs along the way that matter. It's who you become.'

According to Abraham Maslow, the way to feel fulfiled is to have a devotion to something greater than themselves, a vocation. Truth, beauty, goodness, and simplicity, these are not merely attributes to make people feel nice. They are needs that must be fulfiled. Maslow described self-actualization as not something we meet in one great moment like a religious experience. Rather, it involves a process. Let this COVID experience be that experiential process. Quarantine, lockdowns and mandate frustrations. These undertakings allow us to redefine ourselves. Redefine the way we think, the way we feel, and the way we react to circumstance.

The human spirit can never be broken, only become better.

Salud.